STUDIES IN HISTORY, ECONOMICS AND
PUBLIC LAW

Edited by the
FACULTY OF POLITICAL SCIENCE
OF COLUMBIA UNIVERSITY

NUMBER 417

THE AMERICAN MEDICAL PROFESSION
1783 TO 1850

BY
HENRY BURNELL SHAFER

THE AMERICAN MEDICAL PROFESSION
1783 to 1850

BY

HENRY BURNELL SHAFER, Ph.D.

NEW YORK
COLUMBIA UNIVERSITY PRESS
LONDON: P. S. KING & SON, LTD.
1936

Copyright, 1936
BY
Columbia University Press

Printed in the United States of America

TO MY FATHER

GEORGE BURNELL SHAFER

AND MY MOTHER

LOUISE McGINNIS SHAFER

PREFACE

DURING the years from 1783 to 1850, the medical profession was in transition from medieval customs to modern methods. The American medical profession shared in the problems of world medicine. At the same time, it faced the problems of a new and expanding country. This monograph examines medical practices in America during these years and traces the history of the American medical profession. As such, it is concerned with the regular, or allopathic, physician; other practitioners are discussed only incidentally as they impinge upon the development of the regular profession.

For the inception of this work and for scholarly guidance in much of it, I am deeply indebted to Dixon Ryan Fox, formerly Professor of History in Columbia University. After his departure to become president of Union College, Professor John A. Krout generously and helpfully gave his time and attention. I am also indebted to Professor E. B. Greene for many suggestions. Elizabeth Whitney Walther, Chester G. Curtiss and Wade B. Martin gave invaluable advice on the form of the manuscript. Dr. Francis R. Packard, editor of the *Annals of Medical History,* very kindly read the chapter on " The Practice of Physick." Helen C. Wilson has given constant help and encouragement. Naturally, I am fully responsible for any errors which may appear.

For reference material I am especially indebted to the staffs of the library of the Surgeon-General in Washington, D. C., the Philadelphia College of Physicians, the University of Pennsylvania, the Law School of the University of Pennsylvania, the Pennsylvania Historical Society, the New York Academy of Medicine, the New York Historical Society, the Buffalo Historical Society, the Boston Medical Library, the Massachusetts Historical Society, the Berkshire Athenaeum in Pittsfield, Massachusetts, the New York Public Library and the Library of the State of New York.

The section dealing with medical magazines is reprinted here with the permission of the *Annals of Medical History*.

Finally, no list of acknowledgments would be complete without an expression of gratitude to Kata Bokor and Andre Halász. I am indebted to them not only for valuable criticism, but for a friendship without which the preparation of much of this work would have been impossible.

H. B. S.

HADDON HEIGHTS,
24 MAY, 1936.

TABLE OF CONTENTS

	PAGE
PREFACE	7

CHAPTER I
American Medicine at the Close of the Eighteenth Century . . . 11

CHAPTER II
Medical Education . . . 33

CHAPTER III
Medical Education: Studies and Problems . . . 55

CHAPTER IV
The Practice of Physick . . . 96

CHAPTER V
Medical Ethics and Fees . . . 148

CHAPTER VI
Medical Literature . . . 174

CHAPTER VII
Medical Regulations and Societies . . . 200

CHAPTER VIII
Developments in American Medicine . . . 241

BIBLIOGRAPHICAL NOTE . . . 250

INDEX . . . 259

CHAPTER I

AMERICAN MEDICINE AT THE CLOSE OF THE EIGHTEENTH CENTURY

MEDICAL history from 1783 to 1850, both in the United States and Europe, was characterized by transition from medieval and colonial practices of the medical *arts* to the medical *sciences* which we know today. A popular writer on medical history, Howard W. Haggard, has expressed the opinion that:

During the first four decades of the nineteenth century scientific facts were accumulated, methods were developed and the spirit of investigation and observation widely extended. . . . Although medicine advanced greatly as a science during this period, the advances were of no immediate benefit to the patient.[1]

The search for new facts and methods was vindicated between 1840 and 1850 in two great discoveries: the contagious nature of puerperal fever and the anesthetic use of ether. Nevertheless we must bear in mind that physicians during this transition period necessarily relied upon the practices which they had inherited from the past.

Although the revolutionary changes in medicine came after the middle of the nineteenth century, a more scientific attitude on the part of the profession was manifest during the period from 1783 to 1850. New medical schools were established in all parts of the country; books and magazines dealing with medical subjects were published to meet an increasing demand; and there was a notable growth of professional solidarity and criticism engendered by the medical

---

[1] Haggard, H. W., *Devils, Drugs and Doctors* (N. Y., 1929), p. 394.

societies. Standards of medical education improved steadily as the medical schools extended their influence. In some communities the rapid increase in the number of schools resulted in an unwholesome competition for students, but the wide distribution of educational facilities enabled the nation to train the physicians needed to serve a scattered population. During this period hundreds of medical societies were formed, some of which are still in existence, and magazines exclusively devoted to medicine were first introduced to members of the profession.

These developments did not affect all members of the profession at the same time. At the end of the period, therefore, one finds a great contrast between the well-educated and the average practitioner, the latter still relying upon many worthless methods. The very slowness of such changes makes it difficult to point definitely to a given year as the dividing line between the old and the new. Instead we must treat these years as a unit, trace the growth of various institutions and practices, and then call attention to discoveries which were the fruition of the endeavors of the physicians of the period and at the same time were indications of even more far-reaching achievements to follow.

This, briefly, epitomizes the progress of American medicine between the years 1783 and 1850. In the beginning of the period the medical profession was poorly educated; it wrote little either for magazines or regular publications; it was unorganized; and, there was slight regulation of the practice of medicine. In the field of medical theory physicians relied upon previous customs and habits and manifested little of that spirit of scientific inquiry which later came to characterize the profession. In order to understand the changes which did take place we need to survey the medical profession of the United States at the close of the Revolutionary War.

Organized medical education in America has its roots in the colonial period just prior to the Revolution. With the exception of isolated tutorial courses in anatomy and surgery, the formal study of medicine began with the College of Philadelphia, the academic institution which Franklin had founded. Dr. William Shippen, Jr., was interested in establishing a medical school in 1762, but awaited the return of his friend, Dr. John Morgan, who was then studying at his *alma mater*, the University of Edinburgh. Upon the return of Dr. Morgan in 1765, the Pennsylvania Medical School was organized as a branch of the College of Philadelphia. Two years later the college decided upon the rules for attaining the degrees of Bachelor of Medicine and Doctor of Medicine.[2] The school operated until the Revolution interrupted its activities. The revolutionary legislature was hostile to the College of Philadelphia, took away its charter in 1779 and organized the University of the State of Pennsylvania including a medical department as well as the usual liberal arts courses.[3] The College of Philadelphia, including its medical department, continued operation until 1791 when the two medical faculties united as the Medical Department of the University of Pennsylvania. It prospered, especially after 1800, and, despite occasional disturbances which many medical faculties experienced during this period, it became the most influential school in the country.

The two men who were directly responsible for the foundation of the College of Philadelphia Medical School were important practitioners. John Morgan received his early education from Reverend Mr. Finley, an uncle of Benjamin Rush, whose school was attended by the children of prominent Philadelphians at that time.[4] After graduating from

[2] *The University of Pennsylvania* (Phila., 1841), pp. 6-7.
[3] *Ibid.*, pp. 10-11.
[4] *American Museum* (12 volumes, Phila., 1787-1792), VI, pp. 353-355. Rush's article on Morgan is the source of this biographical note.

the College of Philadelphia, Morgan began his medical apprenticeship under Dr. John Redman. He also served as a surgeon with the rank of lieutenant in the French and Indian War. At the conclusion of hostilities on this continent in 1760, he left for Edinburgh to complete his medical education. There he studied with the famous physicians of the time, the two Monroes, Cullen, Rutherford, Whytt and Hope. In London he studied anatomy with William Hunter, an outstanding English surgeon. After completing his work in Edinburgh, he attended lectures in Paris for a winter. While in Paris "he injected a kidney in so curious and elegant a manner that it procured his admission into the Academy of Surgery." During his travels in Europe after his studies, he met Voltaire in Switzerland and Morgagni, a famous Italian physician. Among other honors he was elected to the Royal Society of London, was made a licentiate in the College of Physicians in London, and was elected to the College of Physicians in Edinburgh.

Returning to Philadelphia in 1765, Morgan approached the trustees of the College with a plan for a medical school. His plan was accepted and he himself was elected Professor of Theory and Practice of Medicine. In his " A Discourse upon the Institution of Medical Schools in America; Delivered at a Public Anniversary Commencement held in the College of Philadelphia, May 30 and 31, 1765 " he advanced the plan of education.

The order which I would recommend in the study of Medicine is to begin with Anatomy; then what I have called medical natural History, viz. The Materia Medica and Botany; Chymistry should follow; the Institutes come next; and the study of Practice should compleat the work.[5]

[5] Morgan, John, *A Discourse upon the Institution of Medical Schools in America; Delivered at a Public Anniversary Commencement, held in the College of Philadelphia, May 30 and 31, 1765* (Phila., 1765), p. 16.

This approach to the study of medicine was not put into practice in America until 1849; the medical schools soon fell into an irrational system of requiring students to take the same course of medical lectures in two successive years. The five students, therefore, who received the degree of Bachelor of Medicine in 1769 had not been trained according to Morgan's comprehensive plan of study.

Morgan continued with the school until the outbreak of the Revolution when he became Director-General of the Medical Department, a post which he held for two years before he was forced out by a cabal seemingly headed by William Shippen, Jr. This led to a quarrel which involved Benjamin Rush, Shippen and Morgan of the medical world and many others including Washington, in the political and military circles. In many ways Benjamin Rush was the central character in the quarrel, so it will be discussed later. Morgan spent the years until 1781 working for his vindication. He then returned to his classes at the Medical College, where he remained until his death in 1789.

Unlike Benjamin Rush, Morgan wrote and published few articles. His influence was not in theoretical medicine but in medical education, for he founded a school with principles of sound and careful study. The best estimate of him comes from his friend, Benjamin Rush, who wrote:

He possessed an uncommon capacity for acquiring knowledge. His memory was extensive and accurate; he was intimately acquainted with the Latin and Greek classics. He had read much in medicine. In all his pursuits, he was persevering and indefatigable. He was capable of friendship, and in his intercourse with his patients, discovered the most amiable and exemplary tenderness. I never knew a person who had been attended by him, that did not speak of his sympathy and attention with gratitude and respect.[6]

[6] *American Museum*, VI, p. 354.

Associated with Morgan in the medical school, William Shippen, Jr., also played a commendable part in early medical history.[7] Son of a doctor, he was born into a prominent Pennsylvania family. He too attended Finley's school, but his collegiate degree was taken at Princeton in 1754. The following three years he studied medicine with his father, and then departed for a five-year sojourn in Europe. Although he received his degree from Edinburgh, he spent much time in London where he lived with Dr. John Hunter, studying with Dr. William Hunter and making such valuable friends as Dr. John Fothergill and Mr. William Hewson. After his graduation he visited in France, becoming acquainted with many French physicians.

Having specialized in anatomy and midwifery during his studies, he returned to America resolved to teach these two subjects. He could not have selected phases of medicine less agreeable to his contemporaries. Anatomy, as we shall see later, was taboo, unless pictures and preparations instead of cadavers were used. Fothergill, however, had encouraged Shippen in his decision, and, possibly to further his cause, had given him anatomical plates to present to the Pennsylvania Hospital. The donation made, Shippen began his lectures on anatomy, using a deserted building on his father's place. Fothergill had described him as well-qualified, and to this recommendation as well as to his own ability, his success was due. He did, however, have difficulties with the Philadelphians over the use of cadavers in his lectures.

Midwifery at that time was practiced almost entirely by women, men being called only in exceptional cases. The general attitude persisted that a male accoucheur violated modesty. Shippen set out to practice, and deserves much

[7] Wistar, Caspar, *Eulogium on Doctor William Shippen; Delivered before the College of Physicians of Philadelphia, March, 1809* (Phila., 1818), *passim.*

credit for breaking down ancient prejudice. His pioneer work was long remembered. As late as 1835 Edward Cutbush, speaking at the opening of the Medical Institution of Geneva College, eulogized Shippen when he mentioned the subject of midwifery:

> This is another highly important branch of medical education. Delicacy has thrown a veil around this subject which precludes all remarks before this audience. It may not, however, be improper to state, that Dr. William Shippen of the Philadelphia School, by his suavity of manners and correct deportment, was the first to remove these prejudices, which had long existed in this country, in opposition to male accoucheurs; and I trust that his pupils, and those whom they have instructed, have never violated the laws of strict propriety in their professional intercourse.[8]

After Morgan had presented his plan for the new medical school, Shippen applied to the board of trustees and was elected Professor of Anatomy and Surgery. He continued his work in the school with increasing success and, but for his part in the Revolution, would have had no cloud upon his name. For the moment, it suffices to say that he was accused of bringing about the removal of his old friend, Morgan, from his post as Director-General. Subsequently he himself quarrelled with Rush and finally resigned his post. His standards in the classroom were high; he was an able and exacting teacher, and he stimulated medical students to study and investigation.

The second medical school to be founded in the United States was that of King's College (now Columbia University) with its first session in 1768-1769. In 1770, it conferred upon Samuel Kissam and Robert Tucker the first

---

[8] Cutbush, Edward, *A Discourse delivered at the opening of the Medical Institution of Geneva College . . . February 10, 1835* (Geneva, 1835), p. 9.

degrees of Doctor of Medicine in this country.[9] Unlike Pennsylvania, its history is short and unimpressive. Factions in New York City prevented harmony in any medical school.[10] In 1791 Dr. Nicholas Romayne asked the Regents of the University of the State of New York to take his private medical school under their supervision. Although the Regents granted his request, they felt that favorable legislative action was necessary. As a result a charter was applied for and obtained, but on Columbia's request that it should be given further chance to show its merits the charter was revoked, and Romayne's school was not organized as the College of Physicians and Surgeons until 1807.[11] Columbia continued a haphazard course until its final union with the College of Physicians and Surgeons in 1813. From 1792 until 1810-1811 the total number of students was eight hundred and twenty-three, but the total number of graduates was only twenty-four. In 1810 Pennsylvania graduated almost as many students as attended Columbia.[12] Even after its union with Columbia, the College of Physicians and Surgeons did not effectively use the facilities of the city of New York. Quarrels between the faculty and the trustees

[9] *Cf.* Lane, John E., *Daniel Turner and the First Degree of Doctor of Medicine Conferred by the English Colonies of North America by Yale College, 1723* (N. Y., 1919), p. 367. Turner, however, did not receive his degree as the result of formal study.

[10] The British occupation of New York City throughout the Revolutionary War and the unfortunate burning of the hospital, which had been turned into a barracks for the troops, deterred the development of the medical profession and practice in that city.

[11] Hosack, David, *An Inaugural Discourse at the Opening of the Rutgers Medical College in the City of New York* (N. Y., 1826), pp. 25-27.

[12] *Ibid.*, p. 24. The *Columbia General Catalogue*, 1906 ed., gives the number as fifty-four. This number probably includes the graduates of the College of Physicians and Surgeons which absorbed the Columbia Medical Department in 1813. Hosack was intimately connected with the schools and should have known the correct number.

and among the medical profession in New York City continually hampered its development. Efforts to found new schools, usually under the charter of Rutgers College in New Jersey, did not indicate public confidence in the old school. Its growth was slow, and after the establishment of the Medical Department of the University of the City of New York in 1838, it occupied a secondary position for many years.

The other two medical colleges, which were founded soon after the Revolution, were the Harvard Medical School, commonly called the Massachusetts Medical College, in 1783, and Dartmouth's medical school, under the title of Medical College of New Hampshire, in 1798. By 1800 then there existed four medical schools, two founded in the period immediately prior to the Revolution, and two founded after the Revolution. The schools in Philadelphia and New York could not take care of all the medical students. Undoubtedly some students following the example of Rush and Morgan studied at Edinburgh, but there were few who could afford so expensive an education.

Those who desired medical training, and were unable to attend a medical school, still apprenticed themselves to a doctor in their neighborhood with whom they studied an indeterminate number of years. When sufficient knowledge had been acquired, they assumed the title of doctor and began to practice. An elderly physician writing to a medical journal in 1828 gives us a glimpse of the background of the practitioner who was thus trained during the last decade of the eighteenth century. He frankly stated his difficulties:

I like the monthly report of Diseases in the dispensary very much, the *plan* of it. But 'tis more than I can do to understand it. The names are all new, and for all the knowledge I get of 'em the diseases might just as well be new too, just as well.

I mind just as well when they changed the names of medicines the first time I was plagued in the same way, I never did much in the drug way before, but this change of names fixed me; . . . But I hadn't ought to complain, for the whole country has changed in my time, I mind the revolution; and now there is to be a new President over all and a new Mayor over you. I write sildom and meant to have filled my time and paper with a case . . . for I never saw the inside of a corpse.[13]

It has been estimated that of the thirty-five hundred physicians who were practicing at the outbreak of the Revolution, only two hundred had medical degrees. J. M. Toner, a physician who was interested in medical history, gathered a list of twelve hundred physicians who served in the army during the Revolution. Of these only one hundred had degrees.[14] It does not follow that all were poorly equipped because they had not been to Edinburgh. Many physicians were able men, who were interested in the instruction of their apprentices. Formal education, however, is usually better than informal, and it improved greatly during the first half of the nineteenth century.

The prosperous, interested profession usually publishes and organizes. Before Benjamin Rush began to compile his observations, there was practically no medical publication in America. The first medical treatise was *A Brief Guide in the Small Pox and Measles* published by Thomas Thatcher in Boston in 1677.[15] Occasionally books appeared, but nothing systematic was done. During the first years of the period which we are discussing, Americans relied upon im-

---

[13] *Boston Medical and Surgical Journal* (40 volumes, Boston, 1828-1850), I, p. 799.

[14] Ashburn, P. M., *A History of the Medical Department of the United States Army* (Boston and N. Y., 1929), p. 5.

[15] *Medical Papers Communicated to the Massachusetts Medical Society* ... (Boston, 1790-1850), II, p. 235.

ported English books. Benjamin Rush was the first American to receive national and even international recognition. Especially important were his various volumes of *Medical Observations and Inquiries,* publication of which was begun in 1788. In 1797 the first medical magazine, the *American Medical Repository,* made its appearance under the aegis of Samuel Latham Mitchill.

The absence of medical magazines does not, however, indicate complete indifference to scholarly activities. Physicians contributed articles to the *American Museum,* which ran through twelve volumes from 1787 to 1792. There were frequent disquisitions by physicians on non-medical topics, such as the correspondence between Dr. David Ramsay of Charleston and Dr. Benjamin Rush of Philadelphia tracing the progress of the new Constitution through the state conventions.[16] Many times, too, an ambitious practitioner submitted articles which seem more meterological or agricultural than therapeutical, but it must be remembered that the physician made these studies in order to curb disease at two of its important sources, the air and the soil. Besides Rush, Samuel L. Mitchill, who later founded his own magazine, contributed many articles to the columns of the *American Museum.*

There was more interest in forming medical societies than in publication. An attempt to select the first medical society in the United States carries us back to colonial times. Boston has the best claim. In a letter from Dr. William Douglass of Boston to Dr. Cadwalader Colden of New York City, dated February, 18, 1735-36, the former mentions the organization of the society and its design "to publish some short pieces."[17] The next medical society of which we have

[16] *American Museum,* II.

[17] Burrage, Walter L., *A History of the Massachusetts Medical Society, 1781-1922* (Boston, 1923), p. 1.

evidence is that in New York City. There is a manuscript in the New York Academy of Medicine entitled "An Essay on the nature of ye malignant Pleurisy that proved so remarkably fatal to the inhabitants of Huntington, Long Island; and some other places on Long Island, in the winter of the year 1749, Drawn up at the request of a Weekly Society of Gentlemen in New York, and addressed to them at one of their meetings by Dr. Jno. Bard, New York, 1749." A short-lived society in Philadelphia was created, largely through the efforts of Dr. John Morgan in 1765.[18] These three groups are the local societies which existed in the colonial period. The first provincial society was the New Jersey Medical Society founded at New Brunswick in July, 1766. Through its efforts the first regulatory act was passed in 1772.[19]

Other societies were founded before 1800: the Massachusetts Medical Society in 1781; New Hampshire Medical Society in 1791; and the Connecticut Medical Society in 1792. In 1788 the *American Museum* contained an "*Extract from letter from Dr. Elisha J. Hall, to the president of the Baltimore medical society, on the necessity of passing a law for the regulation of the practice of medicine,*"[20] while a year later there appeared in the same periodical an account of the founding of the Delaware Medical Society.[21] There is evidence of the existence of a "Faculty of Physic" in Charleston as early as 1755, but it was not widely known until David Ramsay became president during the Revolu-

[18] Davis, N. S., *Contributions to the History of the Medical Education and Medical Institutions in the United States, 1776-1876* (Washington, 1877), p. 10.

[19] *New Jersey Medical Society, The Rise, Minutes and Proceedings of ... Established July 23rd, 1766* (Newark, 1875), pp. 3-4.

[20] *American Museum*, V, pp. 25-27.

[21] *Ibid.*, VI, pp. 48-50.

tion.²² A list of its charges for 1792 is in the Boston Medical Library. In Philadelphia the College of Physicians was founded in 1787 with a roll of excellent physicians. Nearly all of these organizations exercised regulatory functions which will be discussed later in this study.

By 1800 the doctors were developing professional morale within their societies. They did not, however, have to rely upon their own organizations for recognition. Able physicians were honored by election to the American Philosophical Society which had been founded in 1743. The roster of the Society for 1768 shows that ten of the forty-eight regular members and twelve of the seventy-three corresponding members were physicians. Of the 1264 members who were elected during the years from 1743 to 1849 two hundred and forty-one were doctors.²³ In New England the American Academy of Arts and Sciences of Boston accorded recognition to the medical profession.

At the conclusion of the Revolution the practice of medicine in the new nation was marked by a widespread reliance upon concoctions of drugs, some of which had been used for centuries in Europe and America. Nevertheless, there was a continuous tendency to simplify prescriptions. The drugs which were most widely used in medicinal compounds included mercury, opium and calomel. Tonics consisted of wines, mercury and other drugs. Bloodletting, purges, emetics and sweating were the common methods of combat-

---

²² McCrady, Edward, *The History of South Carolina under the Royal Government, 1719-1776* (N. Y., 1899), pp. 438-439; Week, Carnes, "David Ramsay, Physician, Patriot and Historian". In: *Annals of Medical History*, N. S. I., No. 5 (N. Y., 1929), pp. 600-607.

²³ American Philosophical Society. *Proceedings...* (Volume II, 1884-1885, Phila., 1885), contains names for 1744 to 1837; and *List of Members of the American Philosophical Society, held at Philadelphia, For Promoting Useful Knowledge* (n. p., n. d.). No elections were held in 1850. Of course, not all physicians were Americans.

ing disease. Perhaps a better approach to the practice of these days is to note what was lacking. Ergot, the drug which was most valuable in childbirth, was unknown in America before 1800. The effective uses of iodine, cinchona bark, morphia and strychnine were not discovered until later.[24] These discoveries, however, were no more significant than the long list of drugs and harmful concoctions which disappeared from the prescriptions of competent physicians.

The use of vaccine, discovered by Jenner in 1796, gradually replaced the practice of inoculation with variolus. Beginning with Shippen, there was progressive improvement in the status of midwifery. The contagious nature of puerperal fever was unknown until Oliver Wendell Homes produced his theory in 1843 and Semmelweiss, working independently in Vienna, demonstrated its truth. Both vacination and the discovery of the contagious nature of puerperal fever were isolated cases of medical progress. They represent no *principle* upon which the profession could act. Many physicians speculated on the causes of disease, but their work antedated the formulation of the germ theory, which later in the nineteenth century was to place medicine upon a more scientific basis.

A great boon to mankind, of which the early physicians were ignorant, was the anesthetic use of ether. Although we shall later discuss medical and surgical practices, we may mention here that the profession avoided surgery whenever possible, or, if forced to resort to it, used bloodletting, intoxication, opium or noise to distract the patient. Whatever advance had been made in surgery during the Revolutionary War seems to have been quickly lost. Within a few decades our surgeons evidently fell below the standard of those who practiced immediately following the war. In 1814 in a

[24] *On the Progress of Recent Science* (N. Y., 1851), pp. 1-23.

review of John Syng Dorsey's book on surgery, the reviewer wrote: "Little can be said in favor of the surgery of our own country, even of the present day. The surgeons formed during the revolutionary war have generally quitted the theatre of action."[25] In the eighteenth century the doctors of medicine practiced dentistry; towards the middle of our period, the dentist and general practitioner parted company.

Returning to the general field of medicine, it may be said that before 1800 the profession relied upon various "systems." The scientific spirit which today we associate with the practice of medicine was lacking. The systems were built up by practitioners who worked out the types of diseases and related them to a part of the body or to natural phenomena. Among these theorists G. E. Stahl, court-physician to the King of Prussia from 1716 to 1734, stressed natural cures. Living in a country with a healthy climate, he observed that his patients threw off disease with comparative ease. Herman Boerhaave, a professor at Leyden University who died in 1738, believed that disease existed in the blood. William Cullen (1710-1790) the Scotsman, stressed the nervous system as the source of disease. Finally, John Brown, at one time a protegé of Cullen, found that specific human ailments resulted from general physical weakness. The supporters of these various systems were inclined to bloodletting, purging and emetics in order to drive out the disorder; then, they rebuilt the body by tonics. The procedure was simple enough, but its simplicity derived from superficial diagnosis.[26]

To a profession which accepted these systems, almost without question, Benjamin Rush came with an inquiring and

[25] *New England Journal of Medicine and Surgery* (15 volumes, Boston, 1812-1826), III, 1814, pp. 190-191.

[26] Rush, Benjamin, *Six Introductory Lectures, to Courses of Lectures upon the Institutes and Practice of Medicine, Delivered in the University of Pennsylvania* (Phila., 1801), pp. 17-22.

critical mind. Naturally he was not alone; Shippen and Morgan have been mentioned, and there were David Ramsay of Charleston, John Warren of Boston, a brother of Dr. Joseph Warren of Bunker Hill fame, and Samuel Bard of New York City. These were able physicians, but none was so influential as Benjamin Rush.

He was born near Philadelphia at Byberry, January 4, 1746.[27] His early education was undertaken by his uncle, Samuel Finley, whose school has been mentioned as the educational institution which Morgan and Shippen attended. Following his graduation from Princeton in 1760 and after considerable hesitation between medicine and the ministry, he apprenticed himself to John Redman, the preceptor of John Morgan, for five and one-half years. In 1766, having received as much as he could from his master, and from Shippen and Morgan, he journeyed to Edinburgh where he studied with the famous physicians of that period, finally coming under the influence of William Cullen. Edinburgh not only gave him a foundation in medicine but also inspired his liberal views concerning penology, politics (in which he became a republican), education, slavery and practically all controversial matters which a Scotch cultural center could discuss. After work in London with William Hunter, he used part of a loan from Benjamin Franklin to visit Paris. In 1769 he returned home to take up the Professorship of Chemistry at the College of Philadelphia, where each of the professors was an Edinburgh graduate.

At that time he found the physicians using bloodletting in pleurisy and rheumatism, but sparingly otherwise; purges and vomits in febrile diseases; and relying principally upon sweating medicines. Boerhaave's theory that the blood was the

[27] Goodman, Nathan G., *Benjamin Rush, Physician and Citizen, 1746-1813* (Phila., 1801), *passim*. Unless other sources are noted this volume is the basis for statements concerning Rush.

MEDICINE OF THE EIGHTEENTH CENTURY 27

source of all diseases was at its height. With his characteristic bluntness, Rush attacked this system and proposed to substitute that of Cullen. His criticism of current medical practices combined with his attacks upon slavery and his radical political ideas brought him into disfavor with the upper classes. He was both popular and active, however, among the poor and in the College.

From 1776 to 1783 the Revolution occupied much of his time. He served in the Continental Congress, signed the Declaration of Independence served in the Medical Department of the army, and succeeded in involving himself in a not too creditable quarrel with Shippen, and, finally, with George Washington. After the Revolution he interested himself in the new Federal Constitution, which he favored, and the new Pennsylvania Constitution. Then he retired from public activity except for writing in the cause of temperance and other reform movements.

It was during his Revolutionary War career that Rush was involved in quarrels having ramifications which included the Conway Cabal to remove Washington and elevate Horatio Gates to the rank of commander-in-chief. The story briefly follows. John Morgan was made Director-General of the Medical Department after the defection of Dr. Benjamin Church. In 1777 William Shippen, Jr., was added to the department in charge of the district west of the Hudson. This step seems to have been part of the machinations to remove Morgan from control and to substitute Shippen. In 1778 Morgan was dismissed without consideration and under a cloud of opprobrium which was not removed until his complete vindication three years later. Shippen appointed Rush director of the Middle States. And then the sparks began to fly.

Rush was shocked by the conditions—and it must be admitted that conditions in any army hospital of 1776 were shocking. At first he protested against the system in letters to Congress and to Washington, but later his ill-will turned against Shippen. Washington, with his usual balance, refused to be drawn into the quarrel and allowed the two doctors to fight the matter out. The result was that Rush's hotheaded attacks defeated their author, and he resigned in 1778. The following year, Shippen was courtmartialed but found not guilty. Rush came to the defence of Morgan in 1781, at his vindication, and Shippen resigned the same year. Although much may be said in favor of Rush's cause, his lack of dignity and his haste undoubtedly weakened his position.

His quarrel with Shippen was notorious enough, but he succeeded in involving himself with Washington to such an extent that a sympathetic biographer is not particularly successful in excusing him. When Rush failed to win Washington over to his point of view, he resorted to an unsigned letter to Patrick Henry in which he cast reflections upon Washington's competence. It is difficult to explain why Rush, who, however impetuous, was certainly straight-forward in his attacks, should have done such a thing. Anyway, Henry sent the letter to Washington, who, by comparing handwriting, easily identified Rush as the author. At that time Thomas Conway with the aid of Charles Lee, Thomas Mifflin and General Gates, was attempting to remove Washington from command. Since Rush was on intimate terms with these men, Washington justifiably concluded that he was party to the plot and remained angry with him for years.

When the work of the Revolution was nearly completed in 1781, Rush returned to his Professorship of Chemistry at the College where he remained (the College merging, in 1791, with the University of Pennsylvania) until his death. After Morgan's death in 1789 he added the Professorship of Theory and Practice of Medicine to his work, and after Adam Kuhn's death in 1796, he also taught physiology. However important his political or reforming career may have been, his greatest interest and his greatest achievements were in the field of medicine.

Rush is not famous for his isolated remedies; rather his contributions are in the encouragement which he gave to scientific inquiry in medicine. We have seen how he came back from Edinburgh as a follower of Cullen, and with what force he set about the demolition of the prevalent theory of Boerhaave. After 1770 he seems to have lost faith in Cullen. For some time he cast about for satisfactory theories, and finally seems to have been influenced by the writings of Thomas Sydenham, who died in 1689, to assume a more scientific attitude. From Sydenham's works, Rush received his general theories and a belief in bloodletting, emetics and purges to reestablish balance in an over-stimulated system.[28]

The essential fact-by-fact approach to medicine, a skeptical attitude toward all comprehensive systems, and a feeling that each theory has some value appear in the following statement from an introductory lecture which he gave on the "Connection between Observation and Reasoning in Medicine:"

A perfect system of medicine may be compared to a house, the different stories of which have been erected by different architects. The illustrious physicians who have been named [Stahl, Boerhaave, Cullen and Brown] have a large claim upon our gratitude, for having, by their great, and successive labours, advanced the building to its present height. It belongs to the present and future generations to place a roof upon it, and thereby to complete the fabric of medicine.[29]

[28] *New York Medical and Philosophical Journal and Review* (3 volumes, 1809-1811, N. Y., 1809-1811), II, p. 83, from Rush's introduction to the *Works of Sydenham* (Phila., 1809).
[29] Rush, *Introductory Lectures*, p. 19.

Over-optimistic as this statement is, it has the breadth which we expect from the scientific mind.

In his address "On the causes which have retarded the Progress of Medicine" he stated many criticisms which aptly applied to medicine of that time, and probably of all time. He said that "indolence and credulity" led physicians to accept systems and statements without sufficient examination. The result for medicine was survival of many manifestly false principles. Again he condemned "the great and unnecessary number of medicines" commonly used and suggested that the content of materia medica could be reduced seventy five per cent. Probably the most significant statement which Rush made was his seventeenth cause: "The neglect to inquire after, and record cures which have been porformed . . . by accidents, or by medicines, administered by quacks, or by the friends of sick people."[30] In other words Rush felt that to fulfill its purpose the medical profession must search out cures and examine all possibilities regardless of their sources.

In one field of medicine Rush made great contributions. Unfettered by tradition, he entered the sphere of mental therapy and brought about a series of reforms. At that time conditions among the insane were unspeakable. Rush in addresses and in his own practice began the so-called moral treatment whereby kindness and occupational therapy were combined to restore sanity. He argued for clean, sanitary buildings and removal from crowded cities to the country where peace and quiet would help restore the patient. He favored segregation of the violent from the passive patients. When he had his patients write down their own symptoms, he seems to have anticipated Freud's mental catharsis, wherein the mentally unbalanced relieve themselves of their complexes by talking about them. All this effort preceded

[30] *Ibid.*, pp. 145-146, 149, 151.

MEDICINE OF THE EIGHTEENTH CENTURY

or was contemporaneous with the work of Philip Pinel, a name of far greater fame in the history of psychiatry.

Rush's most obvious influence upon American medicine came in the yellow fever epidemic of 1793, one of the worst to ravage Philadelphia. Treatments were uniformly unsuccessful until Rush chanced upon an article, addressed to the American Philosophical Society, which he had read years before. In this essay Dr. John Mitchill described how he had treated yellow fever in Virginia in 1737, 1741 and 1743 by giving ten grains of jalap and ten grains of calomel. Rush made it ten grains of calomel and fifteen grains of jalap (adult dose) every six hours until four or five evacuations had taken place. During this time he had the patient drink barley water or chicken broth. After the action of the purge, he let eight or ten ounces of blood, if the pulse were good. As a preventive, he suggested a vegetable diet, exercise and cleanliness. His success with this method was phenomenal, but it caused conflict with part of the public as well as his own profession.

As a result of these quarrels he resigned from the College of Physicians, which he had helped establish, giving a set of Sydenham as a parting gift to prove that his bloodletting practice had the endorsement of that authority. He was attacked in the public prints, and never loath to fight, he returned venom with venom. Finally the quarrel reached the courts in his suit for libel against William Cobbett who had attacked him in the most vicious manner. Winning the suit in 1798, he gave the five-thousand-dollar damages to charity and resumed his practice. However doubtful his contemporaries were of bloodletting, successive generations took up the practice and carried it even further than Rush.

The yellow fever dispute and his law suit were the last of Rush's controversies. As he grew older, his practice declined, but he was always occupied with the poor. A position as Treasurer of the United States Mint enhanced a modest income and he lived comfortably until his death in 1813. He was more fortunate than many leaders, since he lived long enough to see the approval of his efforts by his profession. The memorial ceremonies which the profession held upon hearing of his death amply testify to his national fame.

His medical publications ran to five volumes of *Medical Inquiries and Observations*. His work at the College of Philadelphia and subsequently the University of Pennsylvania brought him in contact with large numbers of medical students, if not a larger number than any other teacher. His influence as the first prolific medical author and the teacher of many prominent practitioners, brought him honors both at home and abroad and gave him a distinction enjoyed by no other American physician throughout this period. Of all his activities he seems to have loved medicine the most, for we find him saying at the time of Shippen's death in 1808:

What that time [death] shall come, I shall relinquish many attractions to life, and among them, a pleasure which to me has no equal in human pursuits. I mean that which I derive from studying, teaching, and practicing medicine.[31]

[31] Slack, Joshua P., *The American Orator*, .. (Trenton, 1815), p. 282.

CHAPTER II

Medical Education

WITH the exception of the four colleges which were founded prior to 1800, formal medical education in the United States began during the first half of the nineteenth century. Throughout this period, the curriculum and requirements changed very little. The years were, however, characterized by an extension of educational facilities in all parts of the nation. Within the schools themselves, there was also improvement in courses and a rise in standards. More significant, the movement for educational reform grew until, by 1850, the profession was well aware of the defects of the medical schools. In this and the following chapter we shall examine the opportunities for medical training, attempt to evaluate them, and trace those developments which gave promise of continued improvement.

EDUCATIONAL REQUIREMENTS

Any young man who desired to become a doctor apprenticed himself for a length of time, usually three years, to some " respectable " practitioner, who thereupon held the title of preceptor. Apparently there were regular charges for this apprenticeship. In the Essex South District of the Massachusetts Medical Society the rates were as follows: for three years advance payment was $150 or at the end of the term $200; for two years advance payment was $120 or at the end of the term $133; for one year advance payment was $65 or at the end of the term $75.[1] David Hosack,

---

[1] Pierson, A. L., Letter Book. Ms. in Boston Medical Library.

a successful physician in New York City, without giving the number of his apprentices or the rates charged, stated that he made $1400 between 1826 and 1829 from his private pupils.[2] In the office of his preceptor the apprentice studied whatever books it contained and did odd jobs. If the doctor was experienced and interested, education in his office might be invaluable; if, on the other hand, the doctor merely wanted an assistant and was himself deficient in education, the training was correspondingly poor. There was neither organized medical reading nor actual practice; with the exception of the three-year requirement, no general rules were drawn up by the profession regulating the training of apprentices before entrance into medical school. In 1837 Robley Dunglison, then a professor in the Jefferson Medical College, provided an outline of reading for medical students. In this he said that the average preceptor placed at the disposal of apprentices his personal library, large or small as the case might be, and then left him to his own devices. Naturally the student followed his own curiosity and failed to lay a broad foundation for medical practice.[3] At all events, this work with the practitioner continued for one year and then was interrupted in each of the following years by a term of at least four months—although at the beginning of the century it was often only three months—of formal study.

Notwithstanding Morgan's proposed curriculum, American schools developed an unique system of medical education. Generally speaking, the *courses* were the subjects which were taught and had the same meaning that the word has today; *lectures* were the daily discussions which the professors gave in their courses; and the *term* meant the period during which all courses were studied. The medical

[2] Hosack, David., List of private pupils educated in the office of . . . from the year 1795 . . . Ms. in New York Academy of Medicine.

[3] Dunglison, Robley, *The Medical Student* (Phila., 1837), p. 126.

men referred to the *term* as a *course of study* or as a *course of lectures* or just as the *lectures* of the professors. The courses which the student took were anatomy, physiology, surgery, a combined course in midwifery and the diseases of women and children, materia medica, theory and practice of medicine, and medical jurisprudence.[4] Now the peculiarity of medical education in America was in the requirement that the student take two terms of these same subjects. In other words, the student took all these courses in his first term, and then returned the next year and repeated the identical courses. The origin of this method in the early years of the medical schools was functional; it arose from the dearth of textbooks and the scarcity of professors, so that only by attending two terms could each student adequately cover each course at least once.[5] As late as 1808 the University of Pennsylvania merely stated that the student desiring a medical degree must attend school for two winters and take each professor's course of lectures.[6] By 1820, however, the practice of requiring a repetition of courses had became universal, for in that year the faculty of the College of Physicians and Surgeons of the City of New York could justify its two-term requirement against the attacks of the medical society of the city by saying, " The graduates of Philadelphia and other medical Colleges in the United States are to attend invariably two courses of every professor."[7] With

[4] *Ibid.*, p. 135 and Catalogs and Circulars listed in bibliography, pp. 253-255. Pennsylvania also had a course in Institutes of Medicine, after 1835, which was an omnibus course, chiefly on medical philosophy.

[5] *American Medical Association, Circular Addressed to Medical Colleges of the United States. By a Committee of the* ... (Phila., 1856).

[6] Minutes of the Medical Faculty. University of Pennsylvania, 1767-1814. 4 volumes. Ms. in Medical School of the University of Pennsylvania, p. 102.

[7] College of Physicians and Surgeons, Minutes of the Meetings of the Faculty of . . . 1811-1815, 1815-1818, 1818-1820, 1820-1823, 1846-1850. Mss. Dean's Office. College of Physicians and Surgeons, p. 191.

the improvement in facilities and the increase in the number of professors the two-term system was continued, and the student merely repeated in his second term the courses of his first.

Since the college requirements were usually more strict than those of the states, we may leave consideration of state laws to a later time.[8] If the medical student did not wish to take the doctorate, he could obtain, in the early years, the degree of Bachelor of Medicine at the end of the first year, or in later years a license to practice medicine. The only exception to the two-term requirement for the degree was made when the candidate had apprenticed himself for four years instead of the usual three, in which case one term of study sufficed. Although there might be variations among the colleges in the length of each term of study or in the number of courses, there were always four general requirements: the candidate must be twenty-one years old; have a good moral character; pass his examinations (the method varying with each institution); and, submit and be examined upon a thesis.

As a basis for comparison with education in Europe, it is interesting to note the requirements at the University of Edinburgh, the institution to which most Americans went for further study. By the requirements of 1767, which were only slightly modified before the general revision of 1833, a student spent three years studying at that or another university. In 1825 this requirement was raised to four years. During these four years, he studied the same subjects as American students. Three months prior to graduation he took an oral examination at the home of a professor; if he was found unsatisfactory in Latin, in literary background or in medicine, he returned to study another year. (This requirement of private examination was dropped in 1811).

[8] *Cf. infra.* Chapter VII on the laws regulating the profession.

Besides passing courses, he submitted a thesis, written in Latin, and was examined upon it. Finally, he was given two hypothetical cases and required to defend his diagnoses before two members of the faculty. From the foundation of the medical school until 1833 all written work was done in Latin; in that year, the use of English was permitted, with the result that in 1840 the last thesis in Latin was presented. At the same time (1833) the student was required to take separate oral and written examinations upon scientific subjects and professional subjects. It is therefore, quite clear why ambitious young Americans often went to Edinburgh for a medical training unobtainable in America.[9]

There was an assumption (though not a rule) that women would not enroll for a medical course. They might qualify as midwives and practical nurses, but the profession and the public at large did not expect them to receive degrees. There was general surprise, therefore, when Elizabeth Blackwell entered Geneva Medical College in 1847 and was graduated in 1849. Although the *Boston Medical and Surgical Journal* was sympathetic and described in detail the actions of Miss Blackwell,[10] others were not so generous. A correspondent of the same journal gave as objections to feminine practice the hardships of the profession, the naturalness of marriage, the nervousness of women and lastly the belief that feminine phrenology proved her unfitted for medicine.[11] The crowning achievement of male logic was reached when the *Ohio Medical and Surgical Journal* asked, in 1848, " If the Almighty did not intend that women should occupy a subordinate place, why in the name of wonder wasn't Adam given to Eve, instead of Eve to

[9] Grant, Sr., Alexander, *The Story of the University of Edinburgh* (2 vols., London, 1884), I, pp. 329-333.
[10] *Boston Medical and Surgical Journal*, XXXVII, p. 405.
[11] *Ibid.*, XLII, pp. 69-75.

Adam?"[12] In 1850 the medical faculty of Harvard admitted a woman to the course, but she withdrew her application. The students

Resolved, That no woman of true delicacy would be willing in the presence of men, to listen to the discussion of the subjects that necessarily come under the consideration of the student of medicine. *Resolved*, That we are not opposed to allowing woman her rights, but do protest against her appearing in places where her presence is calculated to destroy our respect for the modesty and delicacy of her sex.[13]

In Boston and Philadelphia, in the following two years, special institutions were provided for women who wished to become physicians. As matters stood, medical co-education was not an important problem of the profession.

HISTORY OF MEDICAL COLLEGES

We have seen that by 1800, four medical colleges—those of the University of Pennsylvania, Columbia University, Harvard University and Dartmouth College—had been established in the United States. Of these the University of Pennsylvania was by far the largest; three-fourths of all the medical students in the country being in attendance. After 1800, and especially after 1810, medical colleges sprang up wherever there seemed to be sufficient population to support such an institution. A decade-by-decade list of the schools reveals slow development between 1800 and 1810. The College of Physicians and Surgeons of New York City, the Medical Department of the University of Maryland and the

[12] *The Ohio Medical and Surgical Journal* (3 volumes, Columbus, 1848-1850), I, p. 380. For a full account of women in medicine see: Blackwell, Elizabeth, *Pioneer Work in Opening the Medical Profession to Women* (New York, 1895).

[13] New England Female Medical College, Boston, *Annual Catalogue* (Boston, 1851), p. 15.

short-lived Medical Department of Brown University, all were established in 1807.

After the War of 1812, there was a revival of interest reflected in geographical extension, and in new schools for the settled portions of the country. The Medical Department of Yale College, though chartered in 1807, began operation in 1813 and continued without striking results. In New England the only other school was founded at Castleton, Vermont, in 1818. The majority of new schools were in the West. The demand for a college which would be convenient for students from the frontier regions led to the College of Physicians and Surgeons of the Western District at Fairfield, Herkimer County, New York, in 1813. And in 1817 one of the schools destined to play an important role, if a large number of students is any criterion, was chartered at Lexington, Kentucky. This school, the Medical Department of Transylvania University, accomodated the western student, although it yielded to the Medical Institute of Louisville towards the middle of the century. Simultaneously with the Transylvania Medical Department, the Medical College of Ohio was founded at Cincinnati by Daniel Drake (a name which appears often in the history of medical colleges of the Mississippi valley). Drake, however able a doctor he may have been, could not keep a faculty together and the result was his final expulsion. With the possible exception of the South, these colleges provided every section of the country with medical education; but unfortunately the competition of new schools retarded the adoption of higher standards.

During the next decade, the Maine Medical College was organized in connection with Bowdoin College in 1820. In western Massachusetts the physicians petitioned for and founded the Berkshire Medical College with degrees from Williams College. The Medical College of the University of Vermont was founded at the same time. After considerable discussion Jefferson Medical College, arising from the private school of George McClellan, was chartered in 1824 in connection with Jefferson College at Canonsburg, Washington County, Pennsylvania, but was situated in Philadelphia. It was small at first, but after the appointment in 1832, of the popular Granville Pattison, of the University of Maryland, its growth was phenomenal. With its staff and that of the University of Pennsylvania Philadelphia continued to be the medical center of the United States.

Many new schools undertook to meet the need for medical instruction in the South. At the northern edge of the section were the Columbian Medical College in Washington, D. C. (1824) which played little part in medical history and disappeared from the scene for five years (1834-1839), and the Washington College at Baltimore under charter of Washington College, Pennsylvania (1830). Farther south the Medical College of South Carolina (1824) fared little better than the Columbian College, being combined in 1837 with its young rival, the Medical College of the State of South Carolina. Virginia also incorporated its Medical Department in connection with the University in 1828 and by extending the course to nine months called attention to a much needed reform. Georgia in the same year chartered its school.

The mushroom growth of colleges from 1820 to 1830 continued during the next decade. Schools opened their doors at Woodstock, Vermont; Geneva, and Albany in New York; Columbus (Willoughby University), Cleveland and Cincinnati in Ohio. Farther west, the Louisville Medical Institute was founded, beginning lectures in 1839, when it took over the faculty of the medical department of Transylvania University. In the South the Medical Department of the University of Louisiana and a branch of the University of Virginia in Richmond were established. Finally in New York City, the University of the City of New York, after much wrangling, appointed a medical department. The only schools to cease operations were the College of Physicians and Surgeons of Western New York and the Medical College of South Carolina, though the Columbian Medical College and the Medical College of Cincinnati closed temporarily.

During the next ten years the pace was unabated. In the East, the Philadelphia Medical College and the Penn Medical College together with the Woman's Medical College of Pennsylvania and the college for Homeopathy were all opened in Philadelphia. In New York the Medical Department of the University of Buffalo was chartered. In Boston plans for the medical College for women under the auspices of the Female Education Society were completed. Although Ohio and Kentucky refrained from chartering medical schools (the Starling Medical College in Columbus had taken over the Willoughby Medical School), Indiana set up proprietary schools at Evansville, Laporte and Indianapolis. Illinois established similar schools, the Rush Medical College in Chicago, Illinois College and a college at Alton in connection with Shurtleff College which became the College of Physicians and Surgeons of the Upper Mississippi. The University of Michigan organized a medical faculty at the end of the period with its faculty on a salary schedule instead of receiving student fees. Wisconsin, admitted to statehood in 1848, founded its college in Madison. Across the Mississippi, Missouri established schools in St. Louis: the St. Louis Medical Institute, Kemper College (afterwards the Medical Department of the University of Missouri) and Franklin College. In Tennessee, the Memphis Medical Institute, an eclectic school which used only botanic medicines, was founded.

The reasons for this multiplication of schools, in many aspects unnecessary and harmful, were the size of the country, the conditions of the profession and the lack of legislative control. With a population spread over a vast territory lacking adequate means of communication, aspiring students found the journey to eastern centers difficult. Coupled with this difficulty, the belief in sectional diseases and in the influence of climate and soil upon health emphasized the value of medical study in the district where one wished to practice. Also, since the salaries of the professors were paid in student fees and the profession in general did not have large incomes, the doctors were always anxious to start new schools. When either this consideration or quarrels among the members of the faculty did not lead to new institutions, dissatisfaction on the part of groups within the cities or states did. Public distrust of professional monopolies prevented effective legislation in this field. Since the federal government never intervened, anarchy was complete. When the American Medical Association was formed in 1846, one of its first problems was medical education; the Association, however, was voluntary and could gain its ends only by academic cooperation. As medical knowledge increased, longer and more careful study would be required. A gradual elimination of poor schools would follow.

The student had his choice of many schools. The largest in size, those of the University of Pennsylvania, Jefferson Medical College, Harvard and the University of the City of New York, were also the best in the East. In the West, Transylvania led until the Medical Institute of Louisville entered competition. At the end of the period, Rush Medical College with Nathan Smith Davis on its faculty was making progress. Students who were well-to-do could go to Europe. As early as 1802, it is true, the *Medical Repository* boasted "That among the graduates of Edinburgh, . . .

There was not a single one from the United States. The schools of Philadelphia, New York, Cambridge, . . . are engaged in the business of medical education to an extent that is both pleasing and surprising." [14] Nevertheless, many of our best doctors—John W. Francis, Wright Post, Valentine Mott and Jacob Bigelow, Jr.—did go to Europe for further study.

Many medical colleges were associated with academic institutions of higher standards than medical education itself could boast, but that connection was largely nominal. A group of physicians who wished to start a medical school approached a college and asked permission to grant degrees under its charter. Since the medical faculty would not be an expense and might even be financially useful, and since the charters of most colleges allowed them unlimited powers, it was usually easy to obtain this permission. The faculty in these cases considered the school a business. They prescribed the requirements, elected or appointed their own dean, filled the vacancies as they occurred and subject to the laws of the state, gave examinations and granted degrees.

In cases where some real control was exerted by the state, a board of trustees passed upon the regulations of the faculty and by various arrangements approved faculty recommendations. Although in the case of Harvard the medical faculty was almost independent, there was some control exercised by the university authorities. In Pennsylvania the faculty met and passed regulations subject to the trustees of the University. Jefferson, after its separation from Jefferson College in 1827, was placed under the ten Philadelphia trustees who had formerly been appointed to the board of Jefferson College with the medical school as their interest. Transylvania, Ohio and Louisville all worked under the same

[14] *American Medical Repository* (24 volumes, New York, 1797-1824), VI, p. 434.

arrangement. In Vermont, Connecticut and New Hampshire, where delegates from the state medical societies visited and reported on conditions, the medical societies supervised the medical schools.[15] Although the first charter of the College of Physicians and Surgeons of New York City made the entire medical society of the city and county the board of trustees, the number was cut to twenty-one in 1816; and finally in 1826 ten of this number had to be laymen. New York state presented unique control. The Regents of the University of the State of New York had charge of all educational institutions in the state, whether elementary, secondary or collegiate; they appointed the twenty-one trustees and negotiated between the college and the legislature. This system led in 1825 to a quarrel which will be described later. In Maryland the university was controlled by the faculty and regents from 1807 to 1826; in that year trustees were appointed, who after considerable trouble and a lawsuit were again replaced by the faculty and regents in 1839.[16] The college faculty and the state medical society in Connecticut illustrate an harmonious relationship. The society was empowered in 1807 to incorporate a medical college; after negotiations the Medical Department of Yale College was opened in 1813. It will, however, be observed that wherever the trustees were very powerful, friction was sure to develop between them and the faculty; and, on the other hand, in schools where the faculty were all-powerful, its members fell to quarrelling among themselves.

These medical schools were supported largely from student fees. The professors, until the action initiated by the University of Michigan, were not on salary schedules but

[15] American Medical Association, *Transactions* (Phila., 1849), pp. 284-299.

[16] Cordell, E. F., *An Historical Sketch of the University of Maryland School of Medicine, 1807-1890* (Baltimore, 1891), pp. 104, 157.

derived their incomes from the tickets for their lectures. The buildings and equipment were usually furnished by the city or state or by private endowment; thus the College of Physicians and Surgeons received money regularly from the state. New York State treated its medical colleges more liberally than most states; in 1844 it gave Albany and Geneva Medical Colleges $1000 yearly for five years for buildings and equipment, and the Medical Department of University of the City of New York $3000 for one year.[17] Besides this it granted $5000 yearly for three years to Albany Medical College.[18] Hardly a year passed in which this legislature did not make an appropriation of one to three thousand dollars. In addition to direct grants, the legislature approved lotteries in 1809 and 1814; from the first of these the College of Physicians and Surgeons received $5000.[19] The institution in Albany as well as that in Louisville was endowed by the city.[20] In the case of Louisville Medical Institute the city gave $30,000 on the condition that the members of the faculty raise $20,000. This accomplished, the college began its courses in 1839.[21]

Maryland used the lottery extensively to raise funds for its colleges beginning with $40,000 in 1807 and winding up with its last $30,000 in 1826, after a law had been passed abolishing lotteries.[22] In 1828 Maryland also paid the debt

[17] *New York, Laws of ... 1844* (Albany, 1844), pp. 413-414.
[18] Albany Medical College. *Circular, 1844-1845* (Albany, 1844), p. 1.
[19] *New York, Laws of* . . . vol. v, 1807-1809 (Albany, 1809), pp. 439-440; vol. iii, 1812-1815 (Albany, 1815), p. 144.
[20] Albany Medical College. *Circular, 1849-1850* (Albany, 1850).
[21] *Medical Institute of Louisville, Some Account of the Origin and Present Condition of the ... with Remarks on a Late Rejected Report* (Louisville, 1842), pp. 7-8.
[22] *Maryland, Laws of ...* Ed. by Kilty, Harris and Watkins (7 volumes, Annapolis, 1799 for I and no dates for subsequent volumes), sess. 1807, ch. 111; sess. 1811, ch. 132; V, sess. 1813, ch. 125, secs. 5 and 6; V, sess. 1816, ch. 78; *Maryland, Laws of ..*, (Annapolis, 1826), ch. 261.

of the "Faculty of Physic" on its infirmary buildings.[23] At least one other state resorted to the lottery to advance medical education; Kentucky in 1822 authorized a lottery to raise $25,000 for a building for the Medical Department of Transylvania University.[24] Georgia received and sold city lots, and the money, to the extent of $35,000, was invested in the new school.[25] Charles Caldwell, while complaining to the Kentucky legislature about the conditions at Transylvania in 1836, said that the Medical College of Ohio had received $40,000 from the state besides its regular $1600 grant, and that schools in Virginia, Massachusetts and South Carolina regularly received state appropriations.[26] Louisiana helped with a grant of $25,000[27] and the federal government with its cancellation in 1828 of a loan to the Columbian College.[28] Pennsylvania offered little consolation to indebted medical schools, but the legislature did exempt Jefferson Medical College from taxation, the usual taxes to be applied to cut down rent on the college buildings.[29] At Harvard, on the other hand, private endowments continued to enhance the wealth of the school,[30] and in Ohio, Starling Medical College was founded on a grant of $30,000 in 1848 by Lyne Starling.[31] It follows from this discussion that,

[23] *Maryland, Laws of* ... (Annapolis, 1828), ch. 198, sec. 3.
[24] *Kentucky, Acts of* ... (Frankfort, 1823), pp. 149-151.
[25] *Boston Medical and Surgical Journal*, XIX, pp. 63-65.
[26] Caldwell, Charles, *A Report Made to the Legislature of Kentucky on the Medical Department of Transylvania University, February 15, 1836* (Lexington, 1836), p. 30.
[27] *Louisiana, Acts of* ... (New Orleans, 1850), pp. 189-191.
[28] *District of Columbia. Acts of Congress in Relation to ... 1790 to ... 1831* ... Ed. Davis, Wm. A. (Washington City, 1831), pp. 324-325.
[29] *Pennsylvania, Laws of* ... (Harrisburg, 1832), p. 510.
[30] Harrington, T. F., *The Harvard Medical School. A History, Narrative and Documentary, 1782-1905* (3 volumes, New York and Chicago, 1905), III, pp. 439-441.
[31] Starling Medical College. *Catalogue, 1847-1848* (no place), p. 2.

wherever the initial money came from, medical colleges, with the single exception of the University of Michigan, depended largely upon the student fees. This unhealthy condition naturally encouraged profit-making institutions rather than professional schools with high standards of admittance and achievement.

EXPENSE OF MEDICAL EDUCATION

After this brief survey of the medical colleges and their organization, we may return to the prospective student. If his choice was not determined by financial or sectional considerations, how was he to know where he would receive the best medical education? Until Dunglison's *Medical Student* was published in 1837, he had no real guide to the schools, their requirements or faculties, and he had to depend entirely upon such doubtful matter as circulars and advertisements. J. V. C. Smith, in 1839 and again in 1840, partially met this need in his *American Medical Almanac;* and in 1848 another almanac was published in Philadelphia. The college circulars contained information regarding the number of students, graduates, the fees, the requirements, the facilities which the schools offered and often the introductory or commencement addresses. Occasionally these circulars were accompanied by a short history of the school written to arouse public interest rather than to give accurate information. The University of the City of New York listed rates at the boarding houses in order, as it said, to counteract propaganda to the effect that such charges were high in New York City. Nearly all the circulars were accompanied by lists of necessary textbooks. Magazines did not contain such full information in their advertisements and for obvious reasons favored the medical schools in their respective districts. In fact the faculties sometimes published magazines; thus the faculty of the Medical Department of Transylvania University published the *Transylvania Journal of Medicine and Associated Sciences* from 1828 to 1839.

The largest item in the cost of this education was the fee charged per course. Although there was great diversity among the institutions, fees for any one school did not change greatly between 1800 and 1850. Generally speaking rates can be classified according to the location of the school. In the better schools located in the cities, or even at Transylvania which had a good reputation, the rates were high. A large number of institutions such as Jefferson, the University of Missouri, the College of Physicians and Surgeons in the City of New York, Franklin Medical College, Transylvania and the great majority of the schools in the large cities, charged fifteen dollars per course. In Pennsylvania and Maryland (until 1846) the fee was twenty dollars per course, but this was exceptionally high. At the beginning of the period particularly, there was an attempt to differentiate between various courses. At that time chemistry, anatomy and surgery were usually more expensive, but the tendency was toward uniformity in fees.

Some schools charged a set rate for the entire term of study. Woodstock charged forty dollars, Yale seventy-six, Bowdoin forty-five, Columbian College seventy, and Berkshire Medical School fifty-four. The rates, then, varied greatly. One class of schools charged from one hundred to one hundred and twenty dollars and another class, chiefly rural schools, charged around fifty dollars for the entire term.

The needy student was frequently given special consideration. Columbian College allowed one from each state to be designated by the Senators for free attendance.[32] The University of the City of New York allowed ten students upon the payment of twenty dollars each to attend all courses. At

---

[32] *Boston Medical and Surgical Journal*, 1831, p. 615.

Yale the county medical societies could nominate free students, one from each county in Connecticut. In this manner opportunities were afforded the able poor to gain a medical education.[33]

The course or subject fees, however, were not the only charges. Upon entering college a matriculation fee of from three to five dollars was demanded. It was necessary for the student to obtain the tickets or cards of admission to the courses and to register his name upon the school "album." In addition to these fees, there was a graduation or examination fee; thus at Woodstock in 1832 the examination fee was twelve dollars. Most schools, however, included all this in the graduation fee which varied from fifteen dollars in the majority of schools to thirty dollars at the University of Pennsylvania.

Another fee was charged in anatomy courses. This admitted students to the anatomical laboratory where they could further procure at " moderate rates " subjects for dissection. The fee, five or ten dollars as the case might be, went to the demonstrator of anatomy. Students were not always required to take this course; during the early years of the nineteenth century, indeed, the attitude of the public prevented the courses from being properly taught. As early as 1816, however, the faculty of the College of Physicians and Surgeons of New York City changed the anatomical theater into a dissection room;[34] Maryland University required the study of dissection in 1830; and in 1848, according to the American Medical Association report, twenty-five schools demanded such a course before graduation.[35]

[33] American Medical Association. *Transactions*, 1849, pp. 284-299.
[34] Min. of Col. of Phys. and Surg., 1815-1818, p. 100.
[35] For a list of the catalogues upon which this discussion is based see the bibliography, pp. 253-255.

Clinical experience usually required an additional fee of six or eight dollars to the hospitals in which the professors lectured. Many schools saved this expense by providing a school infirmary, dispensary or some similar institution. The fact, however, that the abler surgeons often gave their clinical lectures in the large hospitals placed an additional expense upon city students.

The last item of expenses was board and room which included washing, fuel and incidentals. In the cities this charge seldom exceeded three dollars a week although the lists given on the back pages of the catalog of the University of the City of New York showed some boarding houses for three dollars and fifty cents, and in Louisville the rate was given as from two to four dollars a week. Such rural schools as Woodstock, Berkshire and Fairfield had rates as low as one dollar and twenty-five cents to one dollar and seventy-five cents per week. A poor but enterprising student could follow the example of N. S. Davis who

Like many others *boarded myself,* while in College, living very cheaply, on roast potatoes, pudding and milk, &c., by which I was not only able to pay my way, but saved enough to buy me a small library of books, and a pocket case of instruments, to commence practice with.[86]

These fees do not, of course, cover the cost of the early lectures on anatomy or summer lectures on medicine. These special courses and lectures were additional to the requirements and were conducted for the students who desired more than the mere educational essentials. The cost, nevertheless, of medical education in the United States was not exorbitant. At the University of Pennsylvania, even when it adopted the six-month term, such education could be procured for a sum

[86] French, S. H., *Biographical Sketch of the Medical Department of the the County of Broome* (Binghamton, 1854), pp. 1-2.

not exceeding two hundred and forty dollars per term. At rural schools everything except clothing could be obtained for a sum between one hundred and one hundred and fifty dollars per session.

THE LENGTH OF THE TERM

It is noteworthy that the length of the term, in the first years of the nineteenth century, declined from fourteen weeks at the beginning to thirteen weeks and in some cases even to twelve weeks. The period from 1800 to 1830 was, generally, one of the thirteen-week term; thereafter constant demands by reformers led to the return of the fourteen and even the sixteen-week terms of study. Finally in 1847, the Committee on Education of the American Medical Association recommended a minimum term of six months which was accepted by the College of Physicians and Surgeons and the University of Pennsylvania. A survey of the catalogs of the Vermont Academy of Medicine at Castleton shows the following variation; in 1822 it specified a term of twelve weeks, in 1823, fourteen weeks, in 1824, fifteen weeks, a requirement which lasted until 1833 when the school returned to the fourteen-week term, but by 1844 the standard of sixteen weeks had been attained.

The length of the term in various institutions is discussed in reports by Drs. T. R. Beck, Wendell and Ludlow to the New York Medical Society for 1832 and the American Medical Association Report of 1849.[37] In 1832 only Bowdoin required thirteen weeks, two schools required fourteen weeks, two required fifteen weeks, nine schools sixteen weeks, one school eighteen weeks, the Medical School of the State of South Carolina twenty weeks, and the University of Vir-

[37] Drs. T. R. Beck, Wendell and Ludlow, *Requisitions for Graduation in Various Medical Colleges, Requisitions for Licenses ... States and Territories of the Union, February, 1832*. Chart in the pamphlet collection of the University of Pennsylvania.

ginia ten months. At Virginia, however, the students attended only two lectures daily and the nine-months term (which was the actual length of the term) satisfied the requirement for the degree, whereas at other schools the M. D. requirements included *two* terms of courses. In 1832, the Medical College of Georgia attempted a six-months term; this arrangement lasted five terms, but the school had to give it up.[38] The report of the American Medical Association for 1849 showed that, of the schools reporting, fifteen had sixteen-week terms, five had eighteen weeks, two had twenty, one had eight months, one had nine months (the schools at Winchester and Charlottesville of the University of Virginia), and that the University of Pennsylvania and the College of Physicians and Surgeons of New York City had increased their term to six months. This last action brought a note of commendation from the Alabama Medical Convention in 1847.[39]

We must not, however, dismiss this short term of study without mentioning the attempts to lengthen it. The University of Maryland as early as 1840 and 1841 adopted a six-months term but still allowed pupils to enroll for four months. Beginning in 1843, the Medical Department of the University of the City of New York gave a short course of two months at a cost of fifty dollars. After 1840, most schools opened their anatomical laboratories free of charge to students for one month, usually October, before the regular session. In New England the reading term was developed which required students to read and recite on the phases of medicine. Two of these reading terms, consisting of

---

[38] *Charleston Medical Journal and Review* (3 volumes, Charleston, 1848-1850, Title of I and II: *Southern Journal of Medicine and Pharmacy*), III, p. 392.

[39] *Proceedings of the Medical Convention of the State of Alabama. Held in Mobile, December, 1847*, pp. 5-9.

fifteen weeks each, were given yearly. At Berkshire the fee was twenty dollars per term, and the school required two in connection with each term of courses; thus four reading terms in addition to two terms of regular study were required for the degree, which appreciably raised the educational standard.[40] Other attempts to improve and lengthen the term were made, but mutual suspicion among the schools prevented much action. The reputation of the University of Pennsylvania made it possible for that school to lead the way.

The special schools, which constantly sprang up in connection with regular schools and which merely tutored without granting degrees, increased the length of study. Unfortunately no statistics have come down of the numbers enrolled in these courses. Advertisements for them appeared in the magazines and catalogs. They covered the field of medicine, after the regular session was completed, by means of two lectures a day, during a three- or four-month summer course. The charges ranged from twenty to fifty dollars; in the winter, when there were only reviews, the charge was ten dollars. Among the more famous schools were the Philadelphia school established in 1817 by Dr. P. S. Physick and the Tremont Street School in Boston, founded in 1838 by Drs. Bigelow, Reynolds, Storer and Holmes.[41] In the latter institution a complete course was given, but since the term occupied the summer months, it did not interfere with the regular session. Although its rate of one hundred dollars seems high, the circular stated that " students have no expenses for rent, fuel, lights, attendance, anatomical subjects, and admission to the Hospital and Eye Infirmary." [42]

[40] Berkshire Medical College, *Catalogue*, 1838, pp. 8-9.
[41] Harrington, *op. cit.*, II, pp. 495-502.
[42] Tremont Street Medical School, *Circular, 1847* (Boston, 1847), pp. 3-6.

These schools, in general, rose and fell as certain professors came and went; occasionally they received a charter and became regular collegiate institutions. George McClellan's school in Philadelphia became the Jefferson Medical College, and Nicholas Romayne's school in New York City became the College of Physicians and Surgeons. The value of such extension of the term lay in the opportunity afforded medical students for more organized study. Since the professors in the medical colleges usually conducted these courses, we may infer that the number of students in attendance was large.

To return to the regular session of medical schools, it has been pointed out that there was at least one session during each academic year. Usually it started in early November and lasted until March. If the school had a longer term, the period was from October to April. In some rural institutions such as Woodstock or the College of Physicians and Surgeons of the Western District, the term began in the Spring. Castleton Medical School annually held two terms, which started in late August and late April, and continued a certain number of weeks according to the current regulation. Unless the student attended special and private lectures, he was expected to return to his original preceptor; but many students attached themselves to some one professor and continued their apprenticeship under his guidance.

CHAPTER III

MEDICAL EDUCATION: STUDIES AND PROBLEMS

THE COURSE OF STUDY

THE subjects taught in the various medical schools were, for the most part, the same; anatomy, physiology and chemistry constituted the elementary courses. Advanced work was required in surgery, therapeutics, materia medica, pharmacy, midwifery and diseases of women and children and medical jurisprudence or " forensic medicine." Of these subjects the first three, anatomy, physiology and chemistry, must be fully discussed if the reader is to understand the educational system; the remaining subjects were the foundation of the " practice of physick ", a subject which will be considered separately. We shall mention them here only in analyzing the textbooks which were commonly used.

The history of the courses and the professorships connected with them shows progressive differentiation of subject matter. At the beginning of the period, various subjects were taught in combination. In this manner anatomy, physiology and surgery were often combined; therapeutics, materia medica and pharmacy comprised one course; and midwifery and diseases of women and children and even medical jurisprudence were often grouped together.[1] At the University of Pennsylvania, for example, surgery was separated from anatomy in 1805, but midwifery was

---

[1] Advertisements of colleges in magazines, occasional histories in the catalogs or circulars.

joined with it in 1810. It was not until 1813 that midwifery was given equal standing with the other professorships.[2] This subordinate position of midwifery grew out of the lack of professional status of midwives.

A survey of the entire period reveals a tendency towards more specialized chairs of medicine. The report in 1832 to the New York Medical Society shows that two schools had three professors, two had four, three had five, seven had six, four had seven and only one school the Medical College of Ohio, had eight.[3] By 1849 only one school still had but three professors, and that was the University of Virginia with its longer, nine-month term. Seven schools were reported with six professors, eighteen with seven, two schools with eight, and one, the Medical College of St. Louis, with nine.[4] The constant increase in the number of professorships and the corresponding subdivision of subjects probably indicated improvement in the teaching of medicine.

Anatomy was early recognized as a fundamental requirement in medical instruction. Its study, in America, antedated by at least fifteen years formal medical schools, for the first class in the subject was held by Thomas Cadwalader in Philadelphia as early as 1751; a course in dissection was also conducted from 1752 to 1755 by Dr. William Hunter of Newport, Rhode Island.[5] With the advent of medical schools anatomy, though sharing its position with surgery and physiology, was established as one of the first chairs.

Important as dissection has been for the proper study of anatomy, its use from the days of Vesalius to the twentieth century has required constant effort to circumvent popular

[2] Davis, N. S., *Medical Education, 1776-1876*, pp. 26-27.
[3] Beck, T. R. Wendell and Ludlow, *op. cit.*
[4] A. M. A., *Transactions*, 1849, pp. 284-299.
[5] Davis, *op. cit.*, pp. 11-12.

prejudice. In colonial America the post-mortem was an unusual event. The first one took place in Maryland in 1670 followed by one in Massachusetts in 1675; but the first recorded post-mortem was performed upon Governor Sloughter of New York in 1690.[6] Post-mortems and dissection for medical knowledge are entirely separate in lay minds. Although public sentiment approved the legalization of the post-mortem, popular indignation rose high as soon as the anatomy schools began to use cadavers.

In 1765 riots occurred in Philadelphia against Shippen's school of anatomy. In order to quiet the public, Dr. Shippen published in the *Pennsylvania Gazette* for September 26, 1765 a statement to the effect that he used only bodies of suicides, murderers or cases of special diseases taken from Potter's Field and never took bodies from the church graveyards.[7] Evidently this reply satisfied the mob, for no more trouble occurred for some years.

When public disapproval next appeared, New York City was the scene of the disturbance. During the winter of 1788 students, it appears, dug up bodies "not only of strangers and blacks, . . . but the corpses of some respectable persons," which procedure angered the public. Finally on Sunday, April 13th, a group of small boys playing behind a hospital noticed a human limb hanging out of the window, presumably left there to dry. With the small boy's love of excitement they set about telling people what they had seen, and shortly a large mob gathered to storm the hospital. It succeeded in destroying valuable property, though it failed to get the leg which had caused the trouble;

[6] Hartwell, E. M., "The Hindrances to Anatomical Study in the United States Including a Special Record of the Struggles of our Early Anatomical Teachers" In: *Annals of Anatomy and Surgery* (vol. iii, N. Y., 1881), p. 212.

[7] *Ibid.*, pp. 216-217.

the doctors, whose lives had been threatened by the crowd, were put in jail for their own protection. Excitement subsided only to flare up the next day when the crowd decided to search the homes of the doctors, but they were dissuaded by the combined efforts of the Governor, the Chancellor and the Mayor. Finally in the afternoon the militia had to be called out to prevent the lynching of the doctors imprisoned in the jail, and if a group of " respectable " citizens had not marched to the support of the doctors and fired into the mob, killing three, the affair would have been more serious for the physicians.[8] Rioting broke out the next year in Baltimore. Public hatred of dissectors culminated in the same city when the anatomical theater of Dr. John B. Davidge was destroyed by an incensed mob.[9]

It was in such an atmosphere that the early anatomists and their pupils worked. On the one hand the professors tried to quiet the public by such regulations as that passed by the College of Physicians and Surgeons of the Western District and annually included in its report to the Regents, which stated that " any attempt, proved on a student, to disinter the dead, is punished with expulsion ";[10] or by the somewhat dubious declaration of the faculty of the Vermont Medical College " That bodies disinterred *hereabouts* would not be used in the department of practical anatomy."[11] While the professors were holding off the public, the students were actually engaging in " bodysnatching ", the American equivalent of " resurrectionism ", in an ex-

[8] *American Museum*, III, pp. 389-390.
[9] Hartwell, *op. cit.*, p. 224.
[10] This is in the *Regents' Reports* listed in Bibliography, p. 253.
[11] Putnam, Frederick Wallace Collections. Clippings, circulars, letters, etc. pertaining to Castleton, Berkshire, Vermont, P. & S. Western District and Geneva College. Vermont Medical College folder, pp. 2-3. In the Library of the State of New York, Albany.

asperating fashion. Probably there were a multitude of unknown cases, if we may judge from contemporary reminiscences. Major Butler Goodrich, in Berkshire, threatened to burn the college down unless the practice ended.[12] At Castleton in 1832 after the body of a Hubbardton woman had been stolen from its grave, a mob attacked the medical school and found the headless body. When the head was restored, the crowd was pacified.[13]

Fear that graves would be disturbed led to demands for and the enactment of laws with severe penalties. An enumeration of such laws would include examples from all states. These laws, under some such title as that used in Ohio, "An Act to secure the inviolability of places of human sepulture",[14] carried fines of five hundred to one thousand dollars or jail or both, unless the relatives of the dead person were present or the judge gave permission for post-mortem. The number of laws which were passed is testimony that the professional grave thieves and their competitors and customers, the students, were little deterred by such legislation. Vermont alone passed laws in 1828, 1830, 1832, and even later in that year, apparently without effect.

The first law permitting dissection was passed in Massachusetts in 1649, providing that the bodies of criminals might be used for "Anatomie."[15] In this case dissection seems to have been included to make the punishment more severe. The first law which emphasized the scientific value of dissection was passed by the same state in 1784; this act granted the bodies of those killed in duels or executed for killing in a duel for purposes of dissection.[16]

[12] *The Berkshire Hills* (Pittsfield, 1900-1906), p. 303.
[13] Putnam Collection. *Rutland Herald and Globe* clipping July 21, 1879. This article stated that most bodies came from Albany and Troy.
[14] *Ohio, Laws of*... (Columbus, 1846), pp. 77-78.
[15] *Massachusetts, The Colonial Laws of*... (Boston, 1889), pp. 43 and 139.
[16] Hartwell, *op. cit.*, pp. 211-212.

Shortly after the riots in New York City the state legislature gave judges the right to pass sentence of dissection upon the bodies of murderers, those guilty of arson, and those guilty of burglary.[17] Again in 1790 Congress permitted federal judges to add dissection to the sentences of murderers, and New Jersey passed a similar law in 1796.[18] Evidently the New York legislature granted bodies of convicts dying in prison to the medical profession, for the Columbia faculty commissioned Professors Post and Buchanan to see the Inspectors of the prison.[19] Later the New York legislature awarded the bodies of dead prisoners to other medical schools, as when it gave the college at Fairfield the bodies of all convicts dying in Auburn prison, unless within twenty-four hours they were claimed by friends, relatives or their agents.[20] In 1824 the legislature in Connecticut awarded the bodies of prisoners of Newgate who died without relatives, in addition to those dying by capital punishment, to medical teachers on the condition that the recipients give a one-thousand-dollar bond to limit their dissection to such bodies.[21]

Gradually the public was changing its point of view concerning dissection, but it took the Massachusetts law of 1831 to set an example to other enlightened communities. After defeating the so-called Anatomy Bill of 1830, the legislature reversed itself in 1831 and passed "An Act more effectually to protect the Sepulchres of the Dead, and to

[17] Walsh, J. J., *History of Medicine in New York* (5 volumes, N. Y., 1919), II, p. 389.

[18] Hartwell, *op. cit.*, p. 218.

[19] Minutes of the Faculty of Medicine in Columbia College. Begun February 20, 1792 [to 1808]. Ms. in Dean's Office, College of Physicians and Surgeons.

[20] *New York, Laws of the State of* ... (Vol. V, Albany, 1821), p. 106.

[21] *Connecticut, The Public Laws of the State of* ... (Hartford, 1824), pp. 51-52.

MEDICAL EDUCATION: STUDIES AND PROBLEMS 61

legalize the study of Anatomy in certain cases." It provided that, if any persons, unauthorized by the proper public officials, should dig up or aid in the digging up of bodies, they should be severely punished by fines and imprisonment. Section three states that legally authorized persons could

surrender the dead bodies of such persons, except town paupers, as may be required to be buried at the public expense to any regular physician, duly licensed according to the laws of this Commonwealth, to be by said physicians used for the advancement of anatomical science, preference being always given to the medical schools that now are, or hereafter may be by law established . . . , during such portion of the year as such schools, or either of them, may require subjects for the instruction of medical students: [Provided that no dead body be surrendered if within thirty-six hours anyone wishes to bury it or it is the body of a stranger] so as in no way to outrage public feeling . . . [and the physician should bury the ultimate remains.] [22]

Three years later the law was simplified by granting the boards of health the right to give bodies which might be buried at public expense, unless someone protested.

Following the example of Massachusetts, Connecticut (1833), New Hampshire (1834) and Maine (1844) passed similar laws.[23] Illinois in 1833 reenacted the provision of the act of 1827 providing for dissection of criminals.[24] At the same time that Tennessee relaxed its anti-dissection laws,[25] New York continued to grant the bodies of crim-

[22] *Massachusetts, Laws of* . . . (Vol. III, pt. 2, Boston, 1831), pp. 333-335; *ibid.* (Boston, 1834), pp. 280-282.

[23] *Connecticut, Laws of* . . . (Hartford, 1833), pp. 434-435; *New Hampshire, Laws of* . . . (Concord, 1834), pp. 167-169; *Maine, Acts and Resolves of* . . . (Augusta, 1844), p. 106.

[24] *Illinois, The Revised Laws of* . . . (Vandalia, 1833), p. 203.

[25] Medical Society of the State of Tennessee. *Transactions and Proceedings, 1830-1850* (Nashville, 1830-1850), p. 27.

inals. In the South negroes furnished an easy and, to the whites, unembarrassing source of experimentation. The general attitude of the South, although not recorded in laws, was that of Missouri, which provided that a slave might be dissected with the consent of the owner.[26] Although public opinion was slowly changing, the attitude of a majority outside of the profession was still such as to interfere with the study of practical anatomy.

We have a list of the anatomy text books used by John Warren at Harvard in 1783. They were W. Cheselden's work, first published in 1722, J. B. Winslow's *Anatomical Exposition of the Structure of the Body* published in 1772, and Alexander Monro's *Anatomy of Human Bones, Nerves, and Lacteal Sac and Duct*, published in 1782 at Edinburgh.[27] These works together with J. Barclay's *Nomenclature*, M. Baillie's *Morbid Anatomy* and the works of A. Fyfe sufficed at least until the publication of the three-volume work on anatomy and physiology of the Bell brothers, John and Sir Charles, in 1817, and the two volumes on anatomy by Caspar Wistar of the University of Pennsylvania, in 1811 and 1814. Wistar's work was the first American publication on the subject. W. E. Horner, following what was to become a common American practice, brought it up to date in 1822 and in 1827. When in 1818 the Massachusetts Medical Society listed its required readings for those who wished to take examinations in order to practice, these works of the Bells and Wistar were considered sufficient to cover the study of anatomy.[28]

A large number of translations and modernizations followed these volumes. Xavier Bichat, the famous French

---

[26] *Missouri, Revised Statutes of* ... (St. Louis, 1835), p. 207.

[27] Harrington, *Harvard*, II, p. 7.

[28] *New England Journal of Medicine and Surgery*, VII, pp. 197-198.

physician, was translated by Joseph Togno in 1822 although his work, *General Anatomy applied to Physiology and Medicine* had been published first in Paris in 1801. J. Shaw's *Manual of Anatomy: containing Rules for Displaying the Structure of the Body* . . . was brought to America in 1825 and was quite popular. W. E. Horner struck out on his own in 1826 with a *Treatise on Special and General Anatomy* in two volumes which went through seven editions during the next twenty years. Other favorites of the examining committee of Massachusetts were Carl G. Carus and J. F. Blumenbach, the German physiologist and anatomist, respectively, whose work, first published at Göttingen in 1805, reached English readers in 1827. The textbooks of A. L. Bayle and H. Cloquet were translated from the French.

In 1832 the Massachusetts Medical Society required the *Edinburgh System of Anatomy* and Bell's or Wistar's *System* of the prospective candidate.[29] By 1836 J. Paxton's work on anatomy, issued in England in 1832, appeared in this country and replaced the other English works on the required list.[30] If we add the works of J. Hope the Englishman and H. Cruvelhier, the Frenchman, we have the standard contemporary treatises on class-room anatomy.

These authors in their works discussed comparative, general and pathological anatomy. The first two topics dealt with the skeleton and organs of man in comparison with all animal life and merely named the organs and bones; and the last dealt with the diseased conditions of human organs and was more physiological than anatomical. As the science grew, there was gradual distinction, or indeed divorce, between anatomy and physiology. The text books followed the general order of bones, muscles, organs of sense, hair

[29] Massachusetts Medical Society, *Medical Papers*, V, pp. 70-71.
[30] *Ibid.* (1836), pp. 134-135.

and nails, nervous system, digestive system, respiratory, circulatory system, glands, liver, kidneys, bladder and generative organs. It was an improvement from the Winslow discussion of dry bones, fresh bones, muscles, arteries, veins, nerves, parts of the body, abdomen, thorax and head, but the general outline was still there. As time went on, however, a noticeable improvement took place in the illustrations. In fact the earlier books were devoid of these aids, leaving the student, probably, to rely upon the museums of "wet" and "dry" preparations for his knowledge of the human body. Illustrations became more numerous, until J. Quain's *Human Anatomy*, issued in 1849, contained five hundred drawings.

An examination of the origin of these textbooks shows the dependence of America upon Europe. With the exception of Wistar and Horner, all the books in use were by foreigners. If these were written by Germans or Frenchmen, it may be assumed that they reached America by way of London or Edinburgh, although some, such as Bichat, were translated by Americans. This dependence upon Europe will be seen in other textbooks, but it was greater in anatomy than in other subjects, because the continentals and the English, after 1832, had better chances to develop their methods than American anatomists.

In addition to textbooks, the student had the museums of anatomical preparations. These were plaster casts or bottled preparations developed by some professor and bought by the school, or imported from Europe. It was such a collection which Shippen presented to the Pennsylvania Hospital from Fothergill. The school was usually provided with an anatomical theater in which the professor performed his dissections. Although the students were seated in rising semi-circular rows, the lecture rooms were often so large that those students seated in the back could see very little.

When higher standards developed at the end of the period, this method of instruction was severely criticized.

Very slowly, despite popular opposition, the movement for compulsory practical anatomy to obtain the medical degree made headway, until by 1848 twenty-five schools required it. A demonstrator was in charge of dissection; to him the students paid their fee of five or ten dollars. As the study increased, all schools advertised cadavers for students at "reasonable rates", the Vermont Medical College stating the cost in 1845 at fifteen dollars per subject.[81] It must also be remembered that the many special schools of anatomy connected with the colleges always provided dissection during their short course. The increased practice of dissection is evident in the corresponding increase in the number of guides. Among these one of the most popular was Charles Bell's *System of Dissection explaining the Anatomy of the Human Body, the Manner of Displaying the Parts and their Varieties in Disease*, issued in its first American edition in two volumes at Baltimore in 1814. This was followed by the first American guide by W. E. Horner, *Lessons in Practical Anatomy for the use of Dissectors*. J. Shaw's *Manual of Anatomy* appeared here in 1825, and *The Dublin Dissector*, written by a physician of the Royal College and brought to America in 1835, was used thenceforth. In the next decade the works of Tuson, Parson, Maygrier and Edwards on dissection were made available and used in anatomical laboratories.

From these books, and especially from Horner and E. W. Tuson (edited by Winslow Lewis, Jr.), we get an idea of the contemporary operative procedure in dissection, dress and instruments. Horner, in 1823, prescribed an apron with or without sleeves and advised students to have four knives,

---

[81] Vermont Medical College, *Catalogue*, 1845, p. 10.

a single and double hook, one pair of forceps, one pair of scissors, one blowpipe and two crooked needles.[32] Winslow Lewis, Jr., in his edition, also lists these: scalpels of different forms; a "knife for Myology rounded at the extremity and large", one for blood vessels and nerves, delicate and more pointed; forceps larger than those of American manufacture; medium-size scissors cut well at the point; hooks of chains rather than those which were sold in dissecting cases; a blowpipe; a few curved needles.[33] In addition, he gave a number of rules to lessen the danger to health while working with cadavers; for example, there should be no more fire than is necessary to keep the body from freezing; students should dress warmly, and wear sleeves with rubber wrist-bands; street clothes should never be worn in the anatomy rooms; as soon as bodies were cut up the useless parts should be disposed of; and the student should eat good food and drink a moderate amount of wine to revive the spirits somewhat worn by the fatigue of six lectures and work in the dissecting room.[34] Medical improvement appears in the treatment suggested for cuts and wounds received during dissection. Horner said, while speaking of infection, that

the first intimation of such mischief is the part becoming painful, red, and swollen, and the arm getting somewhat stiff; if in the early stage of these symptoms, a blister be applied accordingly to the recommendation of Dr. Physic, the person live lightly, and take a saline cathartic, the treatment is almost invariably sufficient for the cure.[35]

[32] Horner, W. E., *Lessons in Practical Anatomy for the use of Dissectors* (Phila., 1823), pp. xii-xiii.
[33] Tuson, E. W., *The Dissector's Guide* (Boston, 1844), pp. vii-viii.
[34] *Ibid.*, pp. xi-xii.
[35] Horner, *op. cit.*, p. xxxi.

Lewis, however, advised the application as cauteries of liquid muriate of ammonia or caustic potassium.[36]

Since the bodies were usually cut into five large sections to facilitate dissection, the student could start anywhere.[37] Most of the guides began with the stomach and carefully directed him to the dissection, first of the muscles, and then the organs; from the abdomen, they proceeded to discuss the legs, head and thorax, and upper extremities with regard to muscles, bones, nerves and arteries. Work in this course lasted four or five months, which hardly seems sufficient time to obtain a thorough knowledge of anatomy.

Closely related to anatomy was physiology. The first books usually combined the two studies, and with good reason, for whatever practical study was undertaken included both. Taken as a whole the textbook writers in this field tended to show the differences between organic and inorganic substances, to compare animal with plant life, and to take up the great subdivisions of human life. Again physiology, like anatomy, depended to a great extent upon practical study in the dissection room, and no textbook could ever be a suitable substitute for such activity.

The textbooks used by the early physiology student were A. Haller, *First Lines of Physiology*, translated into English and published at Edinburgh in 1779, and William Cullen's *Institutions of Medicine*, the fourth edition of which was reprinted in Boston in 1788. These two books were replaced by Robert Kerrison's translation of A. Richerand's *Elements of Physiology* and Bichat's work on that subject in 1808 and 1809. J. M. Good and F. Magendie were popular in the 1820's, only to be supplanted by the work of Robley Dunglison (Dunglison was an indefatigable writer

---

[36] Tuson, *op. cit.*, p. xii.
[37] *Ibid.*, p. viii.

of textbooks on every subject except surgery); his work in two volumes ran through eight editions from 1832 to 1856. He was also the only important American writer to be studied on the subject, with the single exception of William Beaumont, whose *Physiology of Digestion* was a genuine contribution to medicine.[38]

Certain books, like most contemporary works, included successive scientific fads. Oliver included his chapter on *Animal Magnetism* not because he believed in it but because he felt that there *might* be something valuable which should be utilized by the regular doctor instead of the quack.[39] Roget's *Outline of Physiology* treated phrenology favorably. On the other hand, most books attempted to give the student a good descripton of the organs and their functions, and paraded no new theories merely for novelty. Those writing at the end of the period, in particular, produced textbooks which were well organized and written with regard to careful teaching.

The study of chemistry underwent great changes — as great if not greater than any other subject. Just prior to 1800 the students were studying P. J. Macquer, R. Watson and A. F. Fourcroy. Of these all were old-fashioned until Fourcroy espoused the teachings of Lavoisier in 1789. The phlogiston theory—a theory which ascribed combustion to a vague element in the atmosphere—had not been supplanted by universal acceptance of oxygen as the element which brings about this phenomenon; the quarrel lasted into the nineteenth century.[40] Lavoisier demonstrated the

---

[38] Other authors of books on physiology in use were J. Muller, W. B. Carpenter and W. S. Kirkes (whose *Hand-Book of Physiology* reached its twenty-first edition in 1908).

[39] Oliver, D., *First Lines of Physiology*... (Boston, 1835), p. vii.

[40] See the *Medical Repository*, 1797-1810 and the articles by Joseph Priestley.

fallacy of the phlogiston theory, and eventually his work replaced all others. W. Henry and H. Davy, two Englishmen, also wrote textbooks improving upon earlier editions. W. T. Brande's *Manual of Chemistry*, subsequently revised by the American, J. W. Webster, was the standard work on chemistry from 1821 to 1840. Although other works were used,[41] the most popular book was that of Benjamin Silliman, Jr., of Yale, which ran through twenty-two editions from 1846 to 1852. It was on every college list and its large publication testifies to its popularity.

These textbooks were always divided into two or three sections. The first was on " imponderable matter " or heat, light, electricity and magnetism; in other words, the first section was really devoted to physics. The ponderable matter included what we now consider the field of chemistry. As time passed, a larger space was devoted to vegetable and animal chemistry under the title of organic chemistry. It was here that rules were given for analysis of fluids which would be useful to a doctor.

It is necessary only to mention briefly the books and courses in the more practical studies. At the beginning of the period, in surgery, the two Coopers, Sir Astley and Samuel, were outstanding authorities. J. S. Dorsey, professor at the University of Pennsylvania and often referred to as the " Father of American Surgery ", brought out, in 1823, his *Elements of Surgery for the Use of Students*. William Gibson, whose book came out in 1827, was very popular. With the decline of Dorsey's work, R. Liston, R. Druitt, A. A. L. M. Velpeau and James Syme, all illustrious foreigners, were used in the American schools with

---

[41] Between 1820 and 1840 J. Murray, E. Turner and Lewis C. Beck, an American, were popular authors on chemistry. From 1840 to 1850, other authors besides Silliman were J. Johnston, T. Graham, A. Gray, G. Fownes and Richard Kane, not one being an American.

or without notes by American teachers; Velpeau in particular was translated and elaborated for the student. Surgery, as time went on, was accompanied as much as possible by clinical instruction in the hospitals of the city or in connection with the schools. The textbooks, with the exception of Valentine Mott's edition of Velpeau, seldom gave much instruction in the preparation of the patient, dressing and bandaging wounds, leaving such matters to practical experience or to the lecturer. Thus the need of clinical instruction was great, but only the larger cities had adequate resources. To make their courses more attractive, the schools often included lists of operations performed in their clinics or hospitals in the catalogs and circulars.

In the course in theory and practice of medicine the general practitioner learned most of what he was to use in later life. The courses usually discussed the diseases common to various sections of the body or followed the broad divisions of fever and finally considered local maladies. In this course the seventeenth century works of Thomas Sydenham and the later writings of Cullen, Herman Boerhaave, Benjamin Rush, the American, and John Hunter (all of the eighteenth century) were studied. William Heberden's *Commentaries on the History and Cure of Diseases* was published in Boston seventeen years after his death, which took place in 1801. J. M. Good, an Englishman, furnished Americans with a four-volume work on general practice, and for the time it was satisfactory. G. Gregory, another Englishman, was introduced to America by Nathaniel Potter and Samuel Colhoun in 1826. Two Americans, James Eberle and W. P. Dewees, of the Jefferson Medical College, published their works in 1830; both were popular, although Eberle's was the better, reaching the fifth edition in 1841. At the same time students were reading William Fordyce and William Tweedie on *Fever* (published in England in 1773 and 1831 respectively), William Stokes on the *Chest* and John Hunter on *Venereal Disease* and *Gun-shot Wounds*. Again Robley Dunglison in 1842 produced two volumes which were exceptionally popular and useful. George Bacon Wood of Philadelphia published a *Treatise on the Practice of Medicine* in two volumes in 1847, which had the distinction of being used as a text by the University of Edinburgh medical faculty.[42] Thomas Watson's *Lectures on the Principles and Practice of Physic* was used with Dunglison and Wood as the textbook at the end of the period. There was, however, a more comprehensive publication by a group of English doctors, the *Cyclopædia of Practical Medicine,* which was introduced to Americans by Robley Dunglison in 1845. It contained a well-organized discussion of the symptoms, causes and treatment of diseases arranged alphabetically and written by specialists on each subject. The authors were not interested in promulgating theories but in presenting accepted cures, and their work represented the best collection of information available at that time.

Indispensable to the theory and practice of medicine was the study of materia medica. At first, W. Lewis, whose *Experimental History of Materia Medica . . .* was first published in London in 1761, was the accepted author on this subject. In 1808, the Massachusetts Medical Society published its pharmacopœia, and J. Murray's *Materia Medica* appeared in New York. Nathaniel Chapman, an American, published his work on the subject in 1817, and the United States was well on its way to develop its own medicinal agents. On January 8, 1817, Lyman Spalding moved that the New York County Medical Society issue a call to medical societies and schools to send representatives to Washington to frame a national pharmacopœia. The meeting

[42] Hartshorne, H., *Memoir of George B. Wood* (Phila., 1880), p. 12.

was held under the chairmanship of S. L. Mitchill, and the *United States Pharmacopœia* resulted in 1820, with the understanding that it was to be revised every ten years.[43] Although Bigelow, of Boston, corrected it to 1822, it was some time before the regular ten-year meetings were carried out. W. P. C. Barton furnished a book on botanic medicines in 1827, two years after the Paris Pharmacopœia was published in New York. The works of J. Pereira and George Bacon Wood and Franklin Bache in their *United States Dispensatory* were general favorites.

The principal guides to the study of midwifery and diseases of women and children, around 1800, were three Englishmen, W. Smellie, who died in 1763, T. Burns and T. Denman. Following these came the work by the American, W. P. Dewees, who published *A Compendious System of Midwifery* in 1824 (which reached its eighth edition in 1837). In 1834 J. Blundell's *Lectures on the Principles and Practices of Midwifery* was made available to American students and was constantly in use. From 1835 until the end of the period the works of C. D. Meigs of Philadelphia, R. Lee, F. H. Ramsbotham, E. Rigby and R. Gooch, the last four being Englishmen, were very popular.

Medical jurisprudence or "forensic medicine" dealt with abortion, poison, rape and other legal phases of the profession and its ethics. T. R. Beck in America provided not only native students but many others with a fine discussion of this subject, for it was translated into German. Prior to this publication the subject was commented upon only incidentally, but Beck's work in 1823 provided a textbook, which revised by his brother J. B. Beck, reached its tenth edition in 1850.[44]

[43] Spalding, James A., *Dr. Lyman Spalding*... (Boston, 1916), p. 283.

[44] Other authors sometimes consulted were W. A. Guy, M. Ryan, A. S. Taylor, S. Traill and J. Chitty, all Englishmen, but none of these seriously threatened the position of Beck's work on college lists.

Such were the textbooks advertised as necessary in the college circulars. In addition, the student had, upon payment of the matriculation fee, access to the college library. These libraries were very small. Although Transylvania had 8000 volumes (or so it advertised) and a few others had between three and five thousand volumes, they were exceptional in the college world. The Medical Department of the University of Buffalo had only 500 volumes in 1846; the Albany Medical College boasted 1822 volumes in 1847; as late as 1839 the College of Physicians and Surgeons of New York City reported only 1200 volumes. Since these were figures for the end of the period, it is obvious that the early years were even leaner in such facilities. The fact that many schools omitted the exact size of their libraries was, perhaps, an indication of the paucity of books. This deficiency characterized the whole country. The first real medical library to be founded seems to have been that of the Pennsylvania Hospital in 1762. In 1788 the College of Physicians of Philadelphia began its library, but in 1858 it had reached only 1000 volumes. The finest medical library in the United States, if not in the world, that of the Surgeon-General in Washington, D. C., was not begun until 1845.

Of the schools which did have libraries, the rules of Harvard for 1816 alone seem to have been preserved. They were: (1) the librarian was in on Tuesday and Saturday between three and five; (2) two books could be taken out at one time; (3) the reservation of books was possible, and renewal of books on "reserve" forbidden; (4) pamphlets could be taken out for one week, octavo or duodecimo for three weeks, and quarto or folio for five weeks; (5) fines on pamphlets were ten cents, octavo fifteen cents and larger volumes were twenty cents per week, any lost book to be replaced after an absence of ten weeks; (6) borrowers had to pay for all damage done; (7) books were to be returned four days preceding the close of the term; (8) borrowers had to pay the fee of $2.00 to the librarian.[45]

GRADUATION

The courses described above constituted a regular term in the medical schools of the United States. The student spent about five or six hours in the lecture room each day during the three, four or more months the particular school was in session.[46] During this time he had daily or weekly quizzes, if we are to believe the requirements listed in the circulars, and finally an examination by the professors. At the end of the first term, he could generally receive a license which was the substitute for the old Bachelor of Medicine degree. This degree was discontinued by the University of Pennsylvania, because few who received it returned to take the M.D.[47] About one-fifth of the students returned to the school, as we have seen before, to study the same courses and to receive the doctorate. It has already been suggested that the reason for this situation was the scarcity of both books and professors in the early years. The increase in professorships and the original requirement of two years' attendance, also, led to the repetition of identical courses. As late as 1808 the faculty of the Medical Department of the University of Pennsylvania stated that students would have to take each professor's course of lectures once, but would have to attend the school for two winters.[48] Gradually two terms of courses, in which the second merely

[45] *Rules for the Library of the Massachusetts Medical College, 1816* (no place, no date), 4 pp.

[46] A. M. A. *Transactions*, 1849, pp. 284-299.

[47] Gould, George M., Ed. *The Jefferson Medical College of Philadelphia* ... (2 volumes, N. Y. and Chicago, 1904), I, p. 18.

[48] Minutes of the Medical Faculty, University of Pennsylvania, 1767-1814, p. 102.

duplicated the first, became the established rule of the schools, and, with the exception of the Ohio Medical Convention's suggestion in 1837, no efforts were made to change it before 1850.

At the end of the second term, the candidate was examined by the professors, individually or collectively, and occasionally by delegates from the state medical society, as the school or state might direct. At that time he also presented and defended a thesis, written in Latin or English, the latter not infrequently faulty. The faculty of Columbia Medical School did appoint committees yearly to make plans for publication of the theses, but the minutes never state whether the school or the student defrayed the cost.[49] This thesis had to be on a medical subject, well written in the student's handwriting and approved by the professors. Transylvania required monographs of from twelve to forty pages.[50] The theses were seldom worthwhile contributions, for they represented performance of duty rather than expressions of true professional interest.

The student's professors harangued him out as they had harangued him in.[51] The addresses introductory to the courses eulogized both the profession and the courses, and advised students on the advantages of study in the institution and on the methods of such study; the commencement addresses were usually of the same type and were highly rhetorical. They revealed a professional tendency to give platitudinous advice. An example is the address to the graduating class of Columbian College in 1827. The orator

[49] Minutes Columbia Medical Faculty, Begun 1792, *passim*. I have examined the theses of the Berkshire Medical College and none of them was printed. This seems to have been voluntary.

[50] *Catalogue of the Medical Department of Transylvania University, 1846-1847*, p. 14.

[51] These addresses are numerous. The University of Pennsylvania Library, particularly, contains an excellent collection of them.

stressed a sacred regard for truth and kindness to the poor. He went on to suggest a proper (and profitable) deportment: "... in your professional intercourse, assiduously cultivate a *pure* and *elevated* style of conversation, *urbanity* and *gentleness* of manner, and *kindness* of heart." Lastly he reviewed those essentials in making a good impression, such as the observance of Sunday, guarding against " infidel sentiments ", temperance and abstinence from gambling and duels.[52] On the other hand, more addresses were occasionally given which stressed the patience a young doctor would need in overcoming popular skepticism concerning new methods.[53] Benjamin Rush in a concluding lecture in 1789 gave sounder advice than was customary. He told the young practitioners who were going to practice in the country to get a small farm in order to win the favor of the people, to get exercise and to furnish occupation during the lax season. Furthermore, he stressed the economic independence which it would give the rural doctor.[54]

Students were now free from their academic labors. In one rural school, at least, old feuds could be forgotten; at Pittsfield the students recalled when they arrived in August and marched through the town, one hundred strong, either for the fun of marching or to pick quarrels with the townsfolk.[55] Sometimes this rowdy spirit was carried too far. At Geneva College, when Miss Blackwell matriculated, it was said that " The rowdy element was so pronounced at

[52] *Boston Medical and Surgical Journal*, I, pp. 673-696.

[53] Ticknor, Luther, *An Annual Address . . . in the Medical Institution of Yale College, January 20, 1841* (New Haven, 1841), pp. 3-4.

[54] Rush, Benjamin, *Medical Inquiries and Observations* (4 volumes, Phila., 1805 and volume v, Phila., 1798), I, pp. 388-390. These were published in installments and also issued in sets at various times.

[55] *People, Scenes and Incidents of Past Days of Pittsfield*. Newspaper clippings in Berkshire Athanaeum, Pittsfield, Massachusetts, pp. 66-67.

MEDICAL EDUCATION: STUDIES AND PROBLEMS

times that there was a strong sentiment in the town to take stringent measures to suppress the school." [56]

Occasionally the townspeople and students gathered in a farewell party, such as the one given at Pittsfield by the friends of the graduates—"after dinner a number of volunteer toasts were drank, which we regret were not preserved—they contained sentiments, happily expressed, favorable to the cause of freedom, of science and religion." [57] The students at Pittsfield expressed their regrets at leaving college in commonplace verse in the local newspaper:

> Go, go, the pleasant hours we part,
> Which like a meteor swiftly flew;
> I bid farewell, it is the last,
> The last, but hearty, fond adieu,
> But, brothers still will meet again,
> In the land where sainted spirits reign.[58]

After graduation and whatever festivals accompanied the commencement exercises, some students returned for graduate study. At least one-fifth to one-fourth of those enrolled in the courses were either graduate doctors or interested laymen. As early as 1793 vain efforts were made to found a graduate school of surgery and midwifery at Columbia.[59] In its report to the Regents for 1839, the College of Physicians and surgeons stated that A. H. Stevens' course at the hospital was free but not to sub-graduates.[60] and later in 1846 it stated that the Spring and Fall courses were given for post-graduate students.[61] For

[56] Putnam Collection, Geneva College, p. 2.
[57] *Pittsfield Sun*, January 8, 1824.
[58] *Ibid.*, December 25, 2823.
[59] Minutes Columbia Faculty, pp. 53-56.
[60] University of the State of New York. *Regents Report*, 1839, pp. 39-41.
[61] New York State. *Senate Documents*, Report 71, pp. 46-47.

the majority of graduates, these courses had no appeal, and they left college prepared to earn their living with whatever information they had garnered in the one or two terms of residence.

DEFECTS OF MEDICAL EDUCATION

Although medical education in the first half of the nineteenth century was improving, its defects were many. The profession in general paid little attention to what was happening in the schools, but such men as Samuel Bard at the beginning of the period and Nathan Smith Davis at its close strove to point out faults and suggest remedies. In the state medical societies efforts were made to raise standards, but the chief ultimate result of all agitation was to lay bare the need for reform, leaving to the American Medical Association the responsibility for correcting the situation. Undoubtedly short terms, poor educational facilities, lack of practical application, support of professors by the fees of students and failure to separate the functions of teaching from those of examination and admittance to the profession were all serious handicaps. But before discussing these defects, it is best to see how quarrels within and among the schools interfered with the attempts to improve education.

The life of Daniel Drake offers a study of medical schools in the West and the difficulties of the profession in that section. Drake was an able, self-made man. Born in New Jersey, he was taken by his family to Kentucky in 1787 when he was two years old. Here he was reared until he was sent to Cincinnati, where he studied with Dr. William Goforth, who had introduced vaccination into the West. After getting his license, he continued his studies and then went to the University of Pennsylvania to receive his M. D. in 1816. The following year he was a professor in Transylvania University but returned to Ohio to agitate for the incorporation of its medical college. With this end accomplished, he began to build up the institution, but by 1822 faculty dissension, centering around his personality, had reduced the faculty to three professors, and he was removed. His own account of his expulsion displays a keen sense of humor, which may have arisen from his great sensitivity to which Mansfield attributes his seeming quarrelsomeness.

After his dismissal, he went to Transylvania in 1824 and remained there until his wife died. In 1830 he was successful at Jefferson Medical College, but decided, in 1835, to revive the Cincinnati College and develop its medical department. Then followed the " War of Extermination " as he called his attempt to ruin the Ohio Medical College and his arch-enemy, John Moorhead. Evidently he was unsuccessful, for he went to Louisville Medical Institute in 1840, where the trustees changed the automatic retiring provision to allow him to stay. He was constantly drawn back to Cincinnati where he attempted to revive the Medical College of Ohio in 1850, but gave it up for two more years in Louisville. In the fall of 1852 he returned again to his first college, and while working hard to rebuild it, broke under the strain. He lived long enough, however, to publish his *Systematic Treatise on the Diseases of the Interior Valley*, which was the result of great labor and an achievement of considerable scope.[62]

[62] This biographical note upon Daniel Drake is based upon the following sources:

To the General Assembly of the State of Ohio (n. d., n. p.), University of Pennsylvania Library.

The following lectures or books by Daniel Drake:

An Anniversary Discourse on the State and Prospects of the Western Museum Society... (Cincinnati, 1820); *An Inaugural Discourse on Medical Education*... (Cincinnati, 1820); *An Introductory Lecture on the Necessity and Value of Professional Industry*... (Lexington, Ky., 1823); *Anniversary Address, Delivered to the School of Literature and*

If Daniel Drake had been an ordinary professor, intent upon self-advancement, there would be no need to include an account of his life and quarrels. But, on the contrary, he was an able physician, anxious to improve the status and knowledge of his profession and to give his pupils a good medical education. In two addresses "An Introductory Lecture on the Necessity and Value of Professional Industry; . . ." and "Strictures on some of the Defects and Infirmities of . . . Students of Medicine", he laid down excellent rules of conduct and study. He told his pupils that they could learn facts only by "protracted labor." Generalizations, he found, are useful, but without sufficient background they lead to the incorporation and dissemination of errors. Finally in this address he advised students constantly to exercise their powers of observation.

In his address on the defects of students, he classified them according to eleven groups, and then proceeded to give advice. Some of it was reiteration, as when he said, "They must learn the great and momentous truth that habits of study can only be acquired by application." His love for his science and his section, however, led him to ask, "Why is it, then, that we continue to look, almost exclusively to our medical brethren on the other side of the Ocean, and not to ourselves for discoveries and improvements?" And

the Arts at Cincinnati (Cincinnati, 1814 [?]); *A Narrative of the Rise and Fall of the Medical College of Ohio* (Cincinnati, 1822); *Discourse on the History, Character, and Prospects of the West* ... (Cincinnati, 1834); *Pioneer Life of Kentucky* ... (Cincinnati, 1870); *Remarks on the Importance of promoting Literary and Social Concert in the Valley of the Mississippi* ... (Cincinnati, 1820); *Strictures on some of the Defects and Infirmities of ... Students of Medicine* (Louisville, 1847); *War of Extermination* (Cincinnati, 1839); *Boston Medical and Surgical Journal*, XX, p. 395; Huettner, Otto, *Daniel Drake and His Followers* (Cincinnati, 1909); Mansfield, E. D., *Memoir of ... Daniel Drake* ... (Cincinnati, 1855).

he answered his own query by saying that, particularly in the West, physicians lacked a professional outlook, were indifferent to the aims of science and did not put forth efforts to investigate ideas and to formulate new ones.

This question regarding our attachment to Europe was not prompted by blatant nationalism. He seems genuinely to have loved the western valley and to have wished to give it an important place in the life of the world. His efforts in behalf of the Commercial Hospital and Eye Infirmary of Cincinnati testify to his public spirit. Our earliest pictures of that city are found in his *Notices of Cincinnati* and *Pictures of Cincinnati*. He lectured constantly upon the Ohio valley, its prospects, how best to develop its cultural background and the need for such facilities as museums. His activities, in medical schools and in the life of his community, probably gave his academic quarrels undue prominence, but in them the unsettled state of medical education was revealed.

The difference between Drake's quarrels in the Ohio Medical School and those in other medical colleges is in the openness with which the disputes were carried on. The deviousness which characterized many such upheavals was emphasized when the *American Medical Recorder* added a postscript to its attack upon the Jefferson Medical College for low standards, in which it said:

We are informed that the whole of the Medical Professors in Jefferson College have been removed; the cause of these proceedings we do not know, but if we were to give an opinion, we should say that a *few* of the old Professors, who no doubt understand that they are to be re-elected, have been at their *old tricks*,—we . . . shall conclude for the present by remarking if elected (pro tem, it can only be) will serve in an institution where confusion, irregularity, and discord have prevailed from the moment of its birth. Eds. Recorder.[63]

But the school did reorganize and go on, a second reorganization taking place in 1839.[64]

A typical medical college controversy was the quarrel in the College of Physicians and Surgeons which reached its climax in 1825 and 1826. The college, at that time, was governed by a board of trustees consisting of the professors and twenty-one members of the medical society of New York City, who were in turn responsible to the Regents of the University of the State of New York. The petty rivalries of the profession in New York City were notorious. Group after group was formed in order to gain control of the medical college, or, failing that, to found a new school. Thus the college was hampered by frequent attempts to found new schools under the Rutgers charter in New Jersey and by the criticism, both fair and otherwise, which was directed against the faculty. We may overlook the earlier attacks and begin with that of 1819 in which the College was charged by the city medical society with setting too high rates, recommending students under twenty-one for the degree, failing to hold public examinations, making false returns of the number of students in order to give an impression of a large enrollment, and quarreling among the faculty.[65]

This attack was overlooked by the Regents, and the school continued as before. Financially it was getting into

[63] *American Medical Recorder* (6 volumes, Phila., 1818-1823), Cont. as: *Medical Recorder of Original Papers from 1823-1830*; resumed old title in volumes XIII, XIV, p. 248.

[64] Holland, J. W., *The Jefferson Medical College of Philadelphia, 1825 to 1908* (Phila., 1908), p. 4.

[65] Faculty of the College of Physicians and Surgeons, Minutes, 1820-1823, pp. 9-19.

such difficulties that in 1822 the professors loaned the college money besides foregoing their share in the examination fee in order to balance the budget. Finally the trustees charged the professors with favoritism, misappropriation of funds and oppression. A Committee of the Regents was appointed in 1825, which, after visiting and inspecting the college, verified the financial difficulties and exonerated the professors of all charges. In addition it proposed that the trustees be increased to twenty-five with nine laymen, six professors and ten trustees from the medical society; thus the laymen would hold the balance of power.[66]

Because of the disputes or because of their desire to play " their old tricks ", the professors resigned in a body, and after various negotiations, some of them secured a charter from Rutgers University for a medical college of which Dr. David Hosack became president. In his inaugural address, Dr. Hosack told the students that the rival faction had offered to allow him to return to the New York school on the condition that he give up a part of one of his departments to the gentleman making the proposal and that another of the resigning group be removed to make room for a member of the opposing fraternity.[67] Immediately after the faculty resigned, applications came in for positions which had been vacated. Hermanus Bleecker, a Regent of the University, was showered with letters of application or letters recommending some candidate for a position.[68]

The results for the College of Physicians and Surgeons are somewhat optimistically stated in the Regents' report to

[66] *Report of a Committee of the Regents of the University Appertaining to the Visit to the College of Physicians and Surgeons in the City of New York* (Albany, 1826), p. 31.

[67] Hosack, *op. cit.*, p. 38.

[68] Hermanus Bleecker Papers. Mss. Library of the State of New York.

the legislature in 1827. They quoted from the report of the Trustees of the College:

'that the College, since its re-organization, has gone into operation with brighter prospects of success in many respects, than have been witnessed in many years. The Professors being now confined to their proper sphere of teaching, have no longer the power, no disposition, to interfere in the government of the College. Thus, discord, suspicion, and strife, have given away to harmony, confidence, and good feeling. The unfortunate state of the college during the last winter, with the circumstance of another Medical School having been established in this city, under the patronage of a College in a neighboring state have had an effect which is to be regretted. To these causes may be ascribed the diminished number of students attending the College at this time.'[69]

Finally, to finish a rather sorry tale, the trustees of the College of Physicians and Surgeons, in reports to the Regents in 1828 and 1829, stated that college debts of $20,000 were held by the former professors. They asked aid from the state to pay this obligation. At the same time they stated that a charter from the state to Rutgers Medical School would further embarrass them financially. Lastly, they stated that the rival professors would use the money which was owed them to run the old school out of business.[70] In a counter-memorial the Rutgers faculty stated that they were unfairly charged, since the Regents' report of 1825 had exonerated them, and went on to say that the superiority of their school *was* driving the old college out of business—a statement not calculated to better the feeling between the two groups.[71]

[69] University of the State of New York. *Regents Report*, 1827, p. 4.
[70] *Report of the Trustees of the College of Physicians and Surgeons of the City of New York, April 4, 1829* (Albany, 1829), pp. 4 and 6.
[71] *Remonstrance of the Rutgers Medical Faculty against the Communication of the Regents Inclosing the Annual Report of the College of*

After 1826 the Rutgers Medical College severed relations with Rutgers University and attempted a connection with Geneva, but it disappeared in 1830.[72] Its students were left to shift for themselves; some at last found refuge at the University of Pennsylvania, which began by refusing any applicant who had done his work at Rutgers, but decided in 1830 to require two terms from these students for which they would pay only one fee.[73] In this manner ended the quarrel which did much to retard New York City's natural development as a great medical center. When the city did develop a large college, it was not the College of Physicians and Surgeons but the Medical Department of the University of the City of New York, on whose staff were some members of the faculty which had resigned at the beginning of the quarrel.

Similar situations threatened the effectiveness of other colleges. In 1832, the Medical College of South Carolina was hopelessly wrecked by the secession of a group which founded the Medical College of the State of South Carolina. Gunning S. Bedford related at a later date the animosity which accompanied this break-up and his uncomfortable position when he arrived in the city to join the faculty of the Medical College of South Carolina. Eventually in 1837, the Medical College of the State of South Carolina absorbed the Medical College of South Carolina.[74] In New England, Castleton and the Medical College of

Physicians and Surgeons of the City of New York, April 4, 1829 (no date), pp. 4 et seq.

[72] *Catalogue of the Rutgers Medical College, 1829-1830*, Pref.

[73] *Minutes Medical Faculty*, University of Pennsylvania, 1828-1845, pp. 65-66, 88.

[74] Bedford, Gunning S., *Address to the Medical College of South-Carolina* (Charleston, 1841), p. 4.

Vermont quarreled over two Canadian pupils.[75] Bowdoin College was under suspicion because of its large number of graduates.[76] Again, when Jefferson Medical College issued a self-laudatory annual announcement in 1834, protests came from Kentucky, Massachusetts and Baltimore.[77] In the late 1840's Jefferson again blundered when it declared that it was not necessary to study in the section in which one was to practice.[78]

And so the story ran. Schools located in the same section were seldom friendly, although Jefferson and Pennsylvania later lived on good terms. Relations between Transylvania and Louisville were most unfriendly after Louisville took the Transylvania faculty in 1839. Until such a state of affairs could be mended, no concerted attack could be made upon the difficulties of medical education, and the status of the schools remained questionable. Eventually improvement might come with the establishment of a number of schools with high standards. Before any such actual move took place there were sporadic attempts to raise the standards. These at least listed the defects in the educational system and tried to eliminate them.

One fault, as we have seen, was the system of supporting professors by student fees. Occasionally the division of proceeds had variations similar to that of the College of Physicians and Surgeons of the Western District, where

[75] Woodward, T., *Hints on the Present State of Medical Education and the Influence of Medical Schools in New England* . . . Pamphlet in collection of the University of Pennsylvania Library.

[76] *Boston Medical Intelligencer* (5 volumes, Boston, 1822-1826), III, p. 59; II, p. 58.

[77] *Boston Medical and Surgical Journal*, XI, p. 118; *Baltimore Medical and Surgical Journal and Review* (1 volume, Balt., 1833-1834), pp. 77-80. Cont. as: *North American Archives of Medical and Surgical Science*, Ed. E. Geddings.

[78] *Northwestern Medical and Surgical Journal* (2 volumes, Chicago and Indianapolis, 1848-1850), I, pp. 457-459.

Each professor collects from the students under him the fee for his ticket: and annually shall receive $200.00 from the treasury of the college, and in case the $200.00 and the fee from his tickets do not amount to the sum of $500.00 anually, then such sum shall be paid him from the treasury, as will make up the sum of $500.00: and wherever the sum of $200.00 and said tickets shall exceed the sum of $800.00 then so much of said sum of $200.00 as shall make up the $800.00 shall be paid out of the treasury; and whenever the tickets shall amount to $800.00 then no money shall be paid out of treasury; but the professor shall receive the tickets only.[79]

Naturally under such a system of payment, it was advantageous to the teacher to have a large enrollment. Jealousy sprang up among the members of the faculty; and unless a school had the standing of the University of Pennsylvania, Jefferson or Harvard, it was difficult to be selective in admitting students. In this connection, too, should be mentioned the candidate's paying the professors for the examination in the event he passed and the professor refunding the money in the event he failed; thus professors were tempted to pass candidates in order to augment their own incomes. The obvious reform of this practice was salaried professors. When such a change was proposed to the committee investigating the College of Physicians and Surgeons in 1825, it feared that "Such a measure would dampen the ardor of literary pursuit in the professors. [It] would take from individuals the proportionate rewards due to their celebrity, and might endanger the ultimate prosperity and success of the institution."[80] With the sole exception of the University of Michigan, all schools continued payment of their professors out of student fees.

[79] Putnam Collection. College of Physicians and Surgeons of the Western District, pp. 4-5. Transcribed from the minutes of the trustees, December 6, 1814.
[80] *Report of the Committee of the Regents, 1825*, pp. 18-19.

Another fault in the system was the repetition of first-term courses in the second. We have already explained the rise of this system in America by the scarcity of textbooks and professors and the manner in which irrational practices escape observation. The failure to divide the courses into elementary and advanced subjects was due to the indifference of the professors, and yet these same men deplored the lack of preparatory training by the students. The preliminary lectures which schools offered undoubtedly lessened this evil, but the only attempt to modify it was made by the University of Michigan, which required candidates for the degree to take examinations in anatomy, materia medica and chemistry at the end of their first term or the beginning of their second.[81]

In order to develop a professional group, it is necessary to have a cultural basis not directly associated with the technical knowledge of the subject. In this respect, medical education was woefully deficient. Although most of the catalogs stated that a knowledge of classical (Latin) language and philosophy was required and that theses must be well written, it is obvious from a survey of the graduates (the catalogs often listed the previous training or degrees of the members of the graduating class) that very few had previous collegiate education. Any attempt on the part of a school to introduce reforms would send students to other schools with lower standards.

Besides these weaknesses, the schools were deficient in provisions for technical training, so essential for all successful scientific work. In the discussion of anatomy, it has been seen that the facilities for dissection were poor. In order to provide practical experience the school organized

[81] Michigan, Medical Department of the University of ... *Preliminary Announcement* (1850), p. 9.

"cliniques" or infirmaries and hospitals, or became associated with city hospitals, in which the student could observe the treatment of cases by the doctor in charge.[82] When the hospitals of Philadelphia refused to permit student attendance, the schools developed school clinics. These were especially useful in the rural colleges where hospitals were rare.[83]

As late as 1849, according to the American Medical Association report, only nine schools had compulsory hospital attendance, nine schools had none and one school (Harvard) reported that attendance was usual. Thirteen schools did not report; among them were such schools as Berkshire, Geneva and other rural schools, and it may be assumed that they did not require this practice.[84] Wherever there was clinical instruction, two criticisms were leveled against it; first, that the professor in charge was inclined to treat and discuss rare diseases instead of the more commonplace diseases which the student would later encounter (a charge which was made by Dunglison in his *Medical Student*);[85] and, second, that the demonstrations in new clinics were practically valueless because the students could not get near enough to the patient for a real examination.[86]

Another criticism of the system grew out of the speed with which students obtained degrees. To most students, professional standards, scientific spirit, the search for knowledge were merely glorified phrases. All they required of

[82] Norris, G. W., *Early History of Medicine in Philadelphia* (Phila., 1886), p. 129, states that the first clinical teaching America was a course given by Dr. Thomas Bond in 1766.

[83] Ware, John, *Discourse on Medical Education* (Boston, 1846), pp. 11-12.

[84] A. M. A. *Transactions*, 1849, pp. 284-299.

[85] Dunglison, *Medical Student*, p. 165.

[86] *Select Medical Library and Bulletin of Medical Science* (6 volumes, Phila., 1841-1846), II, pp. 66-69.

their teachers was a sufficient knowledge to start practice. Even with this beginning, many deserted the profession,[87] which was probably a welcome relief to the general practitioner who found competition for patients too strenuous. As early as 1819, Samuel Bard lamented, " Could we keep out youth at schools until sixteen, at college until twenty, and in the counting house, or at the study of the professions until twenty-four or twenty-five years of age, they would be more generally successful in life." [88]

In 1840 an irate young practitioner, Andrew Boardman, wrote an essay exposing the worst side of medical education. Biased as it was, this essay set forth in all its glaring inefficiency the situation at Geneva College, not one of the best but certainly not one of the worst medical schools of the time. At that college Boardman found students paying for lectures whch they did not attend in order to get a degree from the institution. He found the anatomical amphitheater inadequate for practical demonstration. In a course in therapeutics the professor gave his lecture almost word for word from Eberle's and Dunglison's works, even to Dunglison's poetic quotations. He then contrasted the promises of the circular with what he found. The course in chemistry was not given by a doctor in medicine but by a doctor in divinity; no cadavers were given in anatomy for dissection although the students offered forty dollars for them; the hospital consisted of the second floor of an old building and did not have one operative case.[89]

Such conditions of irregular attendance, easy graduation, due to few requirements and low standards, within the system, account, in part at least, for the tremendous increase

[87] Drake, Daniel, *Strictures on...Students of Medicine*, pp. 13-16.
[88] Bard, S., *Medical Education* (N. Y., 1819), pp. 11-12.
[89] Boardman, Andrew, *An Essay on the Means of Improving Medical Education and Elevating Medical Character* (Phila., 1840), pp. 5-7.

MEDICAL EDUCATION: STUDIES AND PROBLEMS

in the number of graduates of medical colleges. Figures obtained from histories of schools, catalogs of graduates, and from magazines vary to some extent, but the following are sufficiently accurate to show the tendency: 1769-1799, 221; 1800-1809, 343; 1810-1819, 1375; 1820-1829, 4338; 1830-1839, 6849; 1840-1849, 11,128.[90] F. C. Stewart, lecturing in Edinburgh in 1856, stated that there were at that time 5000 medical students per year, of whom 1000 received degrees; and of this thousand only 600 practiced. Considering one physician to every seven hundred persons as an adequate proportion and adding the three hundred foreign doctors who arrived yearly, he still felt that America was under-supplied with physicians.[91] His error was in estimating that only the graduate doctors practiced. Of the others who attended, it cannot be assumed that all were merely curious; many, undoubtedly, received and used licenses as a basis for medical practice, thereby swelling the ranks beyond a reasonable supply. This competition within the profession made it difficult for a doctor to support himself on a truly professional basis. It is noteworthy that such schools as Pennsylvania, Jefferson, Louisville and the University of the City of New York, all with rather high standards, did have enrollments near and over four hundred students.

THE MOVEMENT FOR EDUCATIONAL REFORM

Although there was constant effort toward improvement, most suggestions for change remained buried in addresses to medical societies and introductory and commencement

[90] Clarke, E. H. et al., *A Century of American Medicine, 1776-1876*, p. 359.
[91] Stewart, F. C., *On the Medical Schools and the Conditions of the Medical Profession in the U. S. A.* (Edinburgh, 1856), pp. 111-112. In: *Edinburgh Medical Journal*, August, 1856.

addresses, without effecting any united action. There were, nevertheless, sincere and thoroughgoing reforms attempted. In 1827, the delegates of the New England States and New York, invited by the medical societies of Vermont and New Hampshire to discuss proposals for educational reform,[92] met at Northampton. As a result of their deliberations they resolved: (1) to form a national society; (2) to require the study of medicine for three years after the acquisition of the A.B. degree; (3) to allow only six weeks vacation from preceptorial study; (4) to require one full term of courses; (5) to require two full courses for the M.D.; (6) to insist upon good moral character; and, (7) to put this plan into effect July 4th, 1829.[93]

In 1828 Bowdoin College also suggested a medical convention to discuss means of reform, a suggestion which was accepted by the New York Medical Society.[94] Since the Bowdoin proposal was not even carried out, and the schools seem to have ignored the resolutions of the Northampton meeting, neither of these efforts had any practical results. From Ohio came the next serious attempt at medical improvement. In 1837, the convention of physicians of that state, meeting at Columbus, drew up a series of resolutions and sent them to schools throughout the country. The most important suggestion was that elementary subjects should be studied the first year and more difficult subjects the second year, an attack upon one of the worst features of the educational system.[95]

[92] *Committee of the Massachusetts Medical Society to the Medical Societies of Vermont and New Hampshire* (Boston, 1826), pp. 3-10.

[93] *Proceedings of a Convention of Medical Delegates Held at Northampton in the State of Massachusetts, 1827* (n. p., 1827), 12 pp.

[94] *New York State Medical Society, Transactions of ... 1807-1831* (Albany, 1860), pp. 413-414.

[95] *American Journal of Medical Science* (Phila., 1827-1850), XXII, pp. 526-527.

The most decided movement for educational advancement came from New York State. As early as 1832 the state society collected information upon the requirements, terms and other regulations of the medical schools. In 1838, as a result of a communication from the Onondaga County Medical Society, requesting the appointment of a committee to look into the question of medical instruction, Drs. Manley, Beck and M'Call were appointed. Besides proposing regulations designed to enforce the current laws, the committee suggested that teaching and licensing be separated.[96] The Ely Resolutions, proposed to the same society sometime later, suggested very drastic reforms which included a seven-year study period instead of the prevailing three, a certificate of study by oath, and three years' practice and a six-months term in a hospital for a degree.[97] The Committee felt that the legislative attitude was such that efforts to bring about these reforms in New York State would be futile.[98] Again in 1845, a committee under Nathan Smith Davis offered new resolutions to the New York State Society, chief among which was one proposing that medical societies be given the right to examine students and to expel members.[99]

From New York the fight was taken to the American Medical Association, founded by New York initiative in 1846. Two years later that body accepted the statements and demands made by its committee on education that: (1) all sound medical education be based on clinical and demonstrative teaching; (2) hospitals should open their doors to the colleges; (3) appointments to hospitals should be based

[95] *New York Medical Society, Proceedings of the ... 1838-1840* (Albany, 1840), App., p. 5 and pp. 242-262.
[97] *Ibid., 1844-1846* (Albany, 1846), App. pp. 14-15.
[98] *Ibid.,* App. pp. 16-18.
[99] *Ibid.,* App. pp. 119-129.

upon merit; (4) the demands made in 1847 for a lengthened term of study, higher requirements of admission and others of a similar nature be put into effect; (5) weekly examinations and a certificate of good work in the first term of lectures be required for the second term; (6) the presence of three impartial outsiders be required at the examinations; (7) the thesis be replaced or augmented by five case studies submitted by the student; and (8) the faculty of each school submit a report on its members and its requirements.[100]

Again in 1849 it made further recommendations of which the outstanding additions were the division of the work into two years instead of repetition of the first year, and the establishment of general examining boards conferring certificates from the American Medical Association.[101] Nathan Smith Davis, the chief instigator of the movement, wrote a *History of Medical Education* in 1850 and drove home all the evils of the system with recommended remedies. In this small volume he repeated his points several times, for he realized that only by constant reiteration would the general profession become aware of its needs.

Unfavorable as this picture is, it would be unfair to look back from our vantage point and see only the shortcomings. In 1846, John Watson, perhaps feeling sorry for his profession, declared that there had been an improvement in the general background of medical students, in the extension of the courses of study, by the opening of anatomical laboratories and private courses, in the effectiveness of teaching methods, and in a growing use of hospitals.[102] His

[100] A. M. A. *Transactions, 1848* (Phila. and Balt., 1848), pp. 35-38.
[101] *Ibid., 1849*, pp. 350-352.
[102] Watson, John, *Lectures on Practical Education in Medicine* (n. Y., 1846), pp. 8-18.

estimate of conditions seems to be a fair one. Gradually some of the schools were attempting reforms. The work, too, of the American Medical Association did bring to national attention the state of education and the need for reform, and furnished a valuable forum for discussion. By the end of the period it could no longer be said of the profession that it was ignorant of its own ignorance.

CHAPTER IV

THE PRACTICE OF PHYSICK
GENERAL MEDICINE

We have already seen that the period from the Revolution to 1850 in medical history was marked by a continuation of the transition from the old " systems " in vogue in the eighteenth and earlier centuries to a pragmatic outlook which sought cures for disease and avoided theorizing. In the field of surgery, dentistry was definitely separated from its parent with the foundation of its own schools, magazines and society. Until the discovery of ether and chloroform, surgical improvements were in instruments and performance of difficult operations. Although doctors began the serious study of child-bearing, midwifery profited little with the exception of the introduction of ergot and ether, both of which required experimentation. From a scientific point of view the entire period represents a groping for new and more reliable standards of practice and study; it was essentially a pioneering era in which medicine cut loose from its old concepts and cast about for new principles.

The " fever " theory, the most popular explanation of disease, stated rather vaguely that disease is a result of irritation or excitement. Before rehabilitating a patient by various drugs, it was best to " depress " or calm him. Despite variations in procedure in specific diseases, this general program was followed by a majority of the profession. Schools of physicians were divided according to the phase of the process which they emphasized, a fact pointed out in 1819 by George Sumner of Hartford, who wrote, " When I first came to this place one of the first questions asked, and it was the most common question was, 'Are you a bleeder, or are you a stimulator?'"[1] The usual depressant was bloodletting, which obtained a larger and longer support in America than in Europe. Although many factors, including low standards in our medical schools, tended to prolong the popularity of bleeding, the success of Benjamin Rush in the yellow fever epidemic of 1793, which we have already mentioned, did much to fasten the practice on American medicine.

In treating general fever, bloodletting from the veins (venesection) or arteries (arteriotomy) by means of the lancet was customary. In local affections, which included everything from stomachache to headache, three methods were used, the leech, the cup and the scarifier. The leech, applied to the affected part, sucked its fill and fell off; if an insufficient quantity of blood was lost, hot applications were used to continue the bleeding. Cupping consisted in applying glass vacuums in the same manner as leeches. These cups were of four types: the bell glass shape; the brass mounted glass with a membrane valve; the same with a syringe; and, the brass mounted glass with a stop-cock. In order to create a vacuum the mouth was used to draw out the air; heat was applied or hot sealing wax was placed in the cup. The syringe and particularly the stop-cock were valuable in regulating the flow of blood. When leeches or cups failed to achieve the desired result, or were not used, the skin was lacerated or " scarified." Early scarificators were devices with triangular points which were driven into the skin; the " German spring-lancet " was similar, but added a spring; the more modern instruments had fine cutting blades which, when the spring was released, cut in half circles. Be-

---

[1] Sumner, George, *Sketches of Physicians in Hartford in 1820 and Reminiscences; and in 1837*, by Gordon W. Russell (Hartford, 1890), p. 10.

sides blades, the new instrument had a gauge screw which regulated the depth of the incision.²

The amount of blood extracted depended upon the practice of the physician and the nature of the disease. Although Samuel Gross said that the usual amount was sixteen to twenty-four ounces and that the patients felt cheated if less was extracted,³ most textbooks set the amount at from ten to twelve ounces. The *Cyclopædia of Practical Medicine,* published in America in 1845, said that bloodletting depended upon the heart and pulse but in most cases should be between ten and fourteen ounces, adding that apoplexy required the loss of from forty to fifty ounces.⁴ In 1811 the *Medical Repository* ran the following account:

Depletion seems to have been from first to last, relied upon by Dr. Lucas and the result of the lancet's reiterated application afforded the most ample testimony of its efficacy. The lost of blood sustained by Mr. Niblett was truly astonishing, and we subjoin an account in the words of Dr. L. himself. From the 28th of May to the 26th of July Captain Niblett, (observes Dr. L.) lost by measurement 600 oz. of blood, and by weight 688 drachms—being it is presumed the largest quantity ever drawn from the veins of any human being in the same length of time by medical advice; and for the person to bear it and do well. He was bled fifty different times, and the blood every time was covered with a thick, strong, white coat; and he lost from 4 to 20 oz. each time. He was cupped, and had leeches applied daily for seven weeks, exclusive of bleedings at the arm and the discharge from the seton.⁵

² Maine, Medical Society of the State of. *Journal* (Hallowell, Me., 1834), vol. i, no. 1, p. 38.

³ Gross, S. D., *Autobiography* (Phila., 1887), pp. 152-153.

⁴ *Cyclopædia of Practical Medicine* (4 volumes, Phila., 1845), Ed. by James Forbes, Alexander Tweedie, etc., Rev. Am. Ed. by Robley Dunglison, I, pp. 296-298.

⁵ *Medical Repository*, XIV, pp. 295-296. Since 200 ounces is the amount of blood in the average individual, this seems rather exaggerated.

THE PRACTICE OF PHYSICK

On the other hand, in some cases bloodletting was avoided. At the time of President Harrison's fatal illness his age was given as the excuse for omitting general extraction of blood. Despite occasional attacks, the practice remained the accepted procedure. Remarking upon Gregory's book in 1826, Nathaniel Potter said that Gregory realized that " it is not debility, but disorganization that is to be apprehended in fevers and inflammations." [6]

After bleeding, the body was further evacuated of its ill humors by physicking, sweating, diuretics and emetics. There were three classes of physics, laxatives, purgatives and drastic cathartics. Calomel, a purgative and derivative of mercury, was generally administered in large doses. Seldom, we may hope, did the amount reach that stated in 1843, in the following account:

He compared his sensations to one packed full of beans, stating that he had just taken the eighth of ten doses which had been left for him by a regular physician, a specimen of which he presented. Upon examination, it proved to be calomel; and submitted to the balance weighed sixty grains, the whole of which was then in his stomach as no action had taken place from the organ or bowels.[7]

Murray in his *Materia Medica* recommended as laxatives, manna, tamarind, sulphur and magnesia; for purging, rhubarb (a very popular drug), aloes and bushthorn; and for cathartics, tartis potasse et sodae, muruas sodae and tobacco.[8] The *Cyclopædia* of *Practical Medicine* added sugar, honey, the juice of ripe fruits, malted grain and fermented liquors

---

[6] Gregory, G., *Treatise on the Theory and Practice of Physic*. With notes and addition... by Nathaniel Potter and Samuel Colhoun (2 volumes, Phila., 1826), Pref.

[7] *Boston Medical and Surgical Journal*, XXVII, p. 356.

[8] Murray, J., *Elements of Materia Medica and Pharmacy* (2 volumes in one, Phila., 1808) (6th ed., N. Y., 1834), pp. 14 and 150.

to the list of laxatives; castor oil, gamboge and hellebore root were used as cathartics.[9] In addition to these remedies the Cyclopædia gave the following rules for exhibiting cathartics: (1) to be used in warm rather than in cold climates; (2) to be used in children to bring about regular movements; (3) to be used in melancholy rather than sanguinary temperaments; (4) not to be used too frequently; (5) never to be used when the alimentary canal was inflamed; (6) if quick action was desired, to be used in the morning, but if slow action was preferred, to be given in the evening; (7) the discharge was to be watched even though calomel always colors it.[10] Dissent from this practice is found in Thomas, who as early as 1811 advocated exercise, light diet, gentle laxatives and less frequent bleeding,[11] and also in the *Cyclopædia* which suggested dietary regulation rather than drastic cathartics.[12]

Since evacuation of the bowels was not always considered sufficient to bring about " debility ", emetics were often administered. Among those appearing in Murray were ipecac, squill, tobacco, antimony, sulphate of zinc, sub-acetate of copper and hydro-sulphuretus ammoniac; of these, ipecac was by far the most popular.[13] At a later date the *Cyclopædia* divided emetics into direct, consisting of sulphur of zinc, acetate of copper, carbonate of ammonia and salts of copper all of which acted directly upon the nerves of the stomach, and indirect consisting of all others which had a general effect.[14]

[9] *Cyclopædia*, I, pp. 385-387.
[10] *Ibid.*, I, p. 387.
[11] Thomas, R., *The Modern Practice of Physic* (1st Am. Ed. N. Y., 1811), pp. 25-26.
[12] *Cyclopædia*, I, pp. 481-500.
[13] Murray, *op. cit.*, p. 139.
[14] *Cyclopædia*, II, pp. 780-784.

Besides these major methods of producing debility, the profession sweated the patient by means of mild emetics or it cleansed the kidneys and bladder by inducing urination by means of turpentine, cubebs, potassium iodine and even cantharides.[15] When these failed, balsam and an admixture of calomel and various other combinations probably succeeded. In addition to these medicines, there were a multitude of preparations designed to stimulate menstruation, nasal discharge, salivary discharge and the ejection of matter from the esophagus.

Equally important with bloodletting, physicking and vomiting, the blister, consisting commonly of mustard, was placed upon the affected organ or in a place complementary to it. When the blister was raised, it was pricked and the flow of water was considered efficacious. Dewees, a very practical teacher, gave these directions for the application of blisters: they were to be thick, applied with adhesive tape for twelve hours; before application a thick, hot, drawing poultice, turpentine, spirits of hartshorn, or cayenne pepper and brandy was to be used to arouse the blood and aid the action of the blister; after the application was removed, the blisters, if large, were to be snipped. At times flies were added to increase adhesion, but the author said that they need not be removed, if the skin was dead. If, he continued, further discharge was desired, a basilica ointment or cerate might be applied; on the other hand, inflammation could be reduced by using soft bread and milk or a poultice of fresh hog's lard; and in case of itching, flax seed was very good. He recommended wilted cabbage leaves in cases where other remedies for over-blistering were not available.[16]

[15] *Ibid.*, I, pp. 697-700.
[16] Dewees, W. P., *Practice of Physic* ... (2 volumes, Phila., 1830), I, pp. 41-50.

When the evil humors which caused fever had been removed, the doctor rebuilt the body by means of tonics. Among the most common tonics was mercury. After its introduction into America about 1745, the regular practitioners made much use of it until its ill-effects were noticed, especially by the quacks. An example of its over-use occurred when:

In 1799, W. G. took sixty-four grains by the mouth, 2040 by clyster, and thirty-six hundred grains of triturated mercury were carefully rubbed into his arms and thighs in five days, amounting in the whole to 5704 grains, and the cure was astonishingly rapid.[17]

Other metals listed by Murray as tonics were iron, copper, arsenic, lime and nitric acid; and in the vegetable field he named quinine, gentian, mahogany, oranges and lemons.[18] Besides these wine was generally prescribed. The *Cyclopædia* listed the usual minerals and vegetables, but added iodine in various forms and silver nitrate. It further departed from old medicine by proposing, or rather summing up, various other methods, which would not have been considered earlier in the period, such as cold bathing in moderation and with reason, walking and moderate exercise according to the patient's condition, massage to stimulate the system, and the mental tonic of travel for those who could afford it.[19]

In addition to general prescriptions there were such common stimulants as ether, camphor, opium, musk, ammonia, alcohol and strychnine.[20] Disinfectants came into more use

[17] Massachusetts Medical Society. *Medical Papers*, II, pp. 352 and 418. Paper by John C. Warren.
[18] Murray, *op. cit.*, pp. 93-94.
[19] *Cyclopædia*, IV, pp. 391-404.
[20] Murray, *op. cit.*, pp. 85-92.

as the period progressed with charcoal, chlorine (for gangrene of the lungs), and chlorinated lime and oxide of soda (for ulcers) for human use; for disinfecting in cases of disease, quicklime, charcoal and heat were recommended; and for general use chlorine gas, muriatic and nitrous acids.[21] In case a medicine was needed to act mechanically, an anthelmintic (to remove worms) consisting of iron, olive oil, wormwood, tansey, mercury, and in case of tapeworms, iron filings served the purpose.[22] Murray believed that lithontriptics, such as soda, calx and potassium were useful in dissolving urinary calculi and similar obstructions.[23]

The prescriptions for specific diseases, a century ago, were fulsome combinations of materia medica. The use of prescriptions so complex that it was impossible to isolate the curative factor was an ancient heritage. The following liniment for rickets and muscle strains, compounded by Thomas Sydenham, an eminent authority of the seventeenth century whose writings profoundly influenced Rush, is an excellent example:

Take of the leaves of common wormwood, the lesser centaury, white horehound, germander, ground pine, scordium, common calamint, feverfew, meadow, sasifrage, St. John's Wort, wild thyme, goldenrod, mint, sage rue, cardus benedictus, penny royal, southernwood, camomile, tansey, lily of the valley, all fresh gathered and cut small of each one handful; hog's lard, four pounds; sheep's suet, two pounds; claret, a quart; infuse them together in an earthen vessel upon hot ashes for twelve hours; then boil them till the aqueous moisture is exhaled, and press out the ointment.[24]

[21] *Cyclopædia*, I, pp. 689-695.
[22] Murray, *op. cit.*, p. 214.
[23] *Ibid.*, p. 209.
[24] Sydenham, Thomas, *The Works of* ... (2 volumes, London, 1788), II, p. 135.

This liniment rubbed upon the affected parts in cases of strain was supposed to be helpful. As time passed, the prescriptions became shorter and many of the items mentioned in this prescription disappeared from materia medica, but even at the end of the period, lengthy prescriptions were common.

THE CURE OF SPECIFIC DISEASE

For thousands of years man has suffered from persistent and irritating diseases. Within the last fifty or seventy-five years, some of the more dangerous of these have been eliminated. Many diseases, which today are controlled by preventive medicine, often assumed the proportions of a plague. Other diseases of a common, though less malignant nature, were treated by remedies handed down from one medical generation to the next with gradual additions and with repudiation of old and unsuccessful methods. By this slow growth the profession accumulated a large number of very useful, and, also, a large number of very useless items.

Any study of American diet, or deductions made from observations of foreign travellers upon it, explains the constipation so common among the people. Rich, fried food in copious helpings was consumed at record-breaking speed to the detriment of teeth, digestion and general health. The relation of this diet to nervous headache was recognized by the profession and cathartics " however judiciously administered " were deprecated.[25] This diet with its ill effects upon the general population explains the popularity of Graham and his light diet, for almost any regimen of eating would have been an improvement.

As treatment for constipation, Nathaniel Chapman advised cups or leeches to the spine, daily use of warm baths, rubbing the back and stomach, " mild purgatives " such as

[25] *Baltimore Medical and Surgical Journal and Review*, I, p. 445.

castor oil, daily doses of prunes and charcoal, and mercury as a last resort. In cases of lesions, castor oil, turpentine and croton oil would open the passage, and mustard seed would keep it open. While making these suggestions, he said that a permanent cure could be achieved only by a regular diet of vegetables and fruit, by exercise, avoidance of crackers and similar foods, regular attendance at the stool and " knead the belly for some ten to fifteen minutes." [26] Robley Dunglison, writing soon after the publication of Chapman's article, recommended tobacco in constipation, colic or strangulated hernia, with emetics as relaxants. Enemas were considered helpful.[27] In more severe stomach disorders such as gastritis, Chapman used cold applications and advocated extraction of twenty ounces of blood either by leeches or cups to the abdominal region. When the patient suffered from cancer, he added enemas to keep the bowels open, topical bleeding, blistering and anodynes. Narcotics and sedatives might be used to relieve pain. In other cases of stomach disorder, such as ulcers, he proposed a light diet as the surest remedy.[28]

Gout defied successful treatment. Thomas proposed blisters to reduce the inflammation and wrapping the parts in flannel or "fleecy hosiery." In more common cases he administered rhubarb and opiates, and advised moderate exercise and mild cathartics to prevent recurrence.[29] Much earlier, but certainly summing up medical opinion for this period with regard to gout, Sydenham suggested a proper regimen, exercise and one of his wordy prescriptions which included watercress and horseradish.[30] He also proposed

[26] *American Journal of the Medical Sciences*, XXIII, pp. 99-109.

[27] Dunglison, Robley, *The Practice of Medicine* ... (2 volumes, Phila., 1842), I, pp. 123-124.

[28] See note 26.

[29] Thomas, *op. cit.*, p. 149.

[30] Sydenham, *op. cit.*, II, p. 197.

riding, abstention from wine, one meal daily and avoidance of venery, thus adding the weight of his opinion to the common theory that gout resulted from licentious living.[31] Like gout, rheumatism played its rôle in making people uncomfortable. The common remedies of all diseases were applied, bleeding, purging, sweating and doses of opium; external applications of warm sweet oil were also used in this antiphlogistic system.[32] Dover powders consisting of pulverized ipecac, pulverized opium and sulphate of potassium served as another remedy.[33]

Doctors not only failed to cure consumption, but their treatment of the disease retrogressed from Greek reliance upon sun and fresh air. Nothing positive was done by the physician, and patients remained the victims of quacks who, playing incessantly upon their fears and increasing weakness, offered a worn and feverish system water-cures, steam-cures and every conceivable mixture of useless, though probably harmless, medicines. On the other hand, Sydenham prescribed this remedy: to a solution of one and one-half pounds of sugar boiled until sticky, he added powder of liquorice, elecampane, aniseed and angelica, one-half ounce each; oil of aniseed, two scruples; all this to be mixed and made into troches. His efforts did not stop here, for he added a lolly-pop effect, with liquorice for the stick, composed of two ounces of sweet almond oil, syrup of maidenhair and violets, each one ounce, and enough sugar to give a sticky consistency. For drinking he made a decoction of syrup of white poppies and maidenhair to be taken three times daily.[34] These prescriptions were designed to relieve the cough, and, in cases of pain, to act as a sedative. Ben-

[31] *Ibid.*, II, pp. 216-245.
[32] Dewees, *Practice*, II, pp. 604-606.
[33] *Ibid.*, I, p. 80.
[34] Sydenham, *op. cit.*, II, pp. 472-473.

jamin Rush published an article in 1789 advocating exercise in the open air, but his advice was ignored.[35]

Constant interest of the profession reflects the prevalence of croup among American children. By 1808, according to the *Medical Repository*, Dr. Stearns of Waterford, New York, in an attempt to cure croup had discarded bloodletting and emetics and relied upon calomel and cerated glass of antimony. If the child was two or over, he administered doses of twenty-five or thirty grains of calomel and a corresponding amount of antimony. The article went on to say, " These doses will operate several times by vomit and stool, and generally produce a powerful effect on the disease; if necessary, they are repeated every eight hours, till relief be obtained." [36] The attempt to discard bloodletting failed here as it did elsewhere, and all subsequent medical works suggested bloodletting either at the jugular vein or by means of leeches. Thomas added a light diet and blisters;[37] Eberle approved of warm baths;[38] Dewees, in cases of high temperature, declared that laudanum with antimony was helpful.[39] George B. Wood, towards the end of the period, proposed a somewhat more useful remedy when he put the patient to bed with a flannel next to the skin in order to maintain body temperature. His treatment also included poultices, warm baths, light diet, and the use of the inevitable leeches.[40] A summary of the most common practices in this

[35] Gross, S. D., Ed. *Lives of Eminent American Physicians and Surgeons of the 19th Century* (Phila., 1861), p. 79.

[36] *Medical Repository*, XII, p. 196.

[37] Thomas, *op. cit.*, pp. 114-115.

[38] Eberle, J., *A Treatise on the Practice of Medicine* (2 volumes, Phila., 1830), I, pp. 316-323.

[39] Dewees, *Practice*, I, pp. 358-371.

[40] Wood, G. B., *A Treatise on the Practice of Medicine* (2 volumes, Phila., 1847), I, p. 791.

disease includes warm baths, flannels, reduction of vitality by bloodletting, and laudanum to quiet a high temperature.

Asthma was ascribed in 1826 to impure or smoky air, cold or foggy weather, vapors of lead and arsenic, catarrh, aneurism and organic diseases.[41] About twenty years later the *Cyclopædia* thoroughly summarized the remedies. In the state of paroxysm bloodletting or cupping for congestion in the head were prescribed, leeches, however, were strictly forbidden. When asthma became serious or hysteria set in, opium relieved the patient; for temporary relief, stramonium was prescribed. Other remedies in cases of paroxysm were tobacco, lobelia (a case where the regular practitioners used the universal remedy of the steam doctors), coffee, emetics, nitre and vinegar as refrigerants and lastly a sinapism (mustard plaster) to the feet. In order to prevent recurrence, cold bathing, soap as an expectorant, in more serious cases a change of climate, and a strengthening of general health by bark, steel, oxyde of zinc and bloodletting, were prescribed.[42]

Whooping cough was treated similarly by bleeding, vomiting, purging by castor oil or calomel, and blistering. Following the practice of bleeding near the source of infection, leeches or cups were applied between the shoulders and, if infection spread to the head, to the temples, the blisters being placed between the shoulders. In addition an abstemious diet, which excluded all animal foods and broths, was recommended throughout the illness.[43]

Hydrophobia, another source of constant trouble, received much fruitless consideration. Its cure was never approximated, and the profession foundered in a mire of suggestions which, with a less terrifying disease, would have been amusing. Sydenham took highly rectified spirits of wine to the

[41] Gregory, *op. cit.*, I, p. x.   [42] *Cyclopædia*, I, pp. 219 *et seq.*
[43] Dewees, *Practice*, I, pp. 382-386.

extent of four ounces and mixed it with one ounce of Venice treacle. He bathed the wounded part three times daily with this mixture and during the interim kept it covered with a piece of linen dipped in the concoction.[44] Rush used bloodletting, purging, occasionally adding clysters, sweating and salivation, blisters, cold baths and tonic remedies.[45] Quite useless was the application to the spine of a piece of bar-iron which was then heated. This suggestion was given serious consideration in the *New England Journal of Medicine and Surgery* in 1818.[46]

This array of diseases, for which few cures had been discovered, represented the common ailments of the country. In addition, at intervals plagues swept America, abating only when the seasons changed or when they had run their course. Among these epidemics was one admittedly preventable—smallpox. Before Jenner's discovery of vaccine, the profession (during the years we are discussing) relied upon inoculation. Vaccination and inoculation may be distinguished as follows: vaccination is the introduction of cowpox whereas inoculation is the introduction of the actual smallpox matter. Since few states made either inoculation or vaccination mandatory, universal protection was impossible. Once a patient contracted the disease, he was given a light diet and mild laxatives. Although Sydenham considered fresh air better than letting blood, Gregory, while agreeing with him, said that many doctors did not. Finally Gregory gave opiates when the pustules were nearing maturation to prevent the patient's scratching himself.[47]

[44] Sydenham, *op. cit.*, II, p. 468.

[45] Rush, Benjamin, *Medical Inquiries and Observations* (5 volumes, Phila., 1798), V, pp. 227-236.

[46] *New England Journal of Medicine and Surgery*, VII, p. 37.

[47] A discussion of laws relating to vaccination will be found in Chapter VII, pp. 216-217; Sydenham, *op. cit.*, II, pp. 58-71; Gregory, *op. cit.*, pp. 190-193.

Twenty years after the signing of the Declaration of Independence, cow-pox vaccine was used by Jenner. It is generally accepted that Benjamin Waterhouse introduced vaccine into America in 1800. Another claim, however, appears in a letter dated Ipswich, 13 January, 1829, from Thomas Manning to A. L. Pierson, probably of Boston, in which he stated:

> by 2 spring ships from London in 1800 I rec'd from a brother Dr. I. C. Manning then in London persuing medical research vaccine virus direct from Dr. Woodvilles small pox vaccine institution, in 2 several parcels not accompanying each other the first on thread and 2nd on ye points of six inoculating lancets, by ye thread, I communicated ye disease, the lancets failed, in ye summer & autumn of 1800. I vaccinated more than 100 persons[,] also furnished Dr Fisher[,] Waterhouse & other Medical gentlemen with vaccine virus some gentlemen were repeated supplied; several of my vaccine patients were the same autumn fully tested by repeated small pox inoculations with recent small pox matter and exposed to several small pox patients having the disease by inoculation; by authority granted by this town for the express purpose of testing the efficiency of vaccine virus; my vaccine patients in every instance resisted the small pox.[48]

This is just another of those difficult, but more or less academic, questions of priority in any enterprise. What is important is that vaccine was proven successful, and its use spread with considerable rapidity throughout the country. Examples of faith in the new treatment would probably be many, but that of Josiah Bartlett of Boston, who vaccinated his two sons in 1802 and exposed them to smallpox for twenty days in order to give public proof of the value of

---

[48] Pierson, A. L., Letter Book, Ms. in Boston Medical Library.

vaccination, shows the lengths to which physicians would go to prove the efficacy of such a discovery.[49]

The general theory that all diseases derived from fever leads one into an involved discussion. The failure of the profession to cure yellow fever, the attempts of the seaports to safeguard their commercial interests by showing that ships from infected ports did not introduce the disease—these facts together with its frequent appearance in such large cities as New York, Philadelphia and New Orleans during the summer months, led the profession to look for its source in the communities where it appeared. A melancholy search through history caused E. H. Smith to see great similarity between yellow fever and the plague of Athens. In a long series of articles in the *Medical Repository,* he dwelt upon these similarities and finally concluded:

If local causes originated a pestilence in Athens, local causes may generate a Yellow Fever in Philadelphia and New York. To these, then, be our attention more scrupulously directed; and let us be more solicitous in the inspection of our houses, yards, streets and docks, than of cottons and woollens, of vessels from the West-Indies and ships from the Mediterranean.[50]

At the same time, 1798, the College of Physicians of Philadelphia suggested in a letter to Thomas Mifflin, then governor of Pennsylvania, that the city be cleaned up, that dangerous ships be unloaded at a distance from the city, that the sewers be closed, that the filth be removed daily and that no more alleys or narrow streets be built. The Academy accepted the prevalent belief that the disease was not contagious but in the local atmosphere.[51] All of these suggestions were

[49] Bartlett, Josiah, *An Historical Sketch of the Progress of Medical Science in the Commonwealth of Massachusetts* (Boston, 1813), pp. 19-20.
[50] *Medical Repository*, II, p. 104.
[51] *Ibid.*, II, pp. 329-331.

timely, and if the municipalities had followed them carefully and had set up efficient health boards or rejuvenated those in existence, much that was done many years later in Havana and the Canal Zone might have been accomplished at this early period in the United States.

Although yellow fever was constantly considered from the point of view of prevention, efforts were made to cure it as well as other fevers. In a general prescription for fevers, Dewees listed common remedies for lessening temperature, such as cool air and cooling drinks, blistering in the locality of the fever (or, in case it was general, at the extremities), bleeding, purging and sweating.[52] Rush's famous treatment of yellow fever by purging with ten grains of calomel and letting ten ounces of blood set a record of cure which left a definite impression upon American medical procedure. Gregory, in a different method, proposed warm water, camomile or eupatorium tea to induce vomiting. He then settled the stomach by a wine-glassful of lime water and milk, twenty drops of turpentine and ten grains of carbonate of potash in a spoonful of lemon juice or a tablespoonful of vinegar every two hours; and eight or ten drops of laudanum in peppermint to quiet the patient. He followed the usual procedure of poultices to the stomach and occasionally to the feet; a teaspoonful of charcoal every hour was an excellent disinfectant; lastly, soda water and iced lemonade relieved the temperature. It is interesting to note that he did not follow Rush's use of bloodletting in this fever, a fact no doubt due to his English background.[53]

Although yellow fever spread such terror that many people hurriedly left the affected centers for the suburbs whenever it made its appearance, it was an American disease with which the people were familiar. Cholera Asiatic, unlike

---

[52] Dewees, *Practice*, I, pp. 64-88.
[53] Gregory, *op. cit.*, I, pp. 150-151.

other forms of cholera, was known only by the tales of its horror in Europe. When it was spreading throughout Europe, in 1832, and when it made its appearance in America shortly after, the medical profession cooperated to prevent its development. Committees were formed in the various cities to study the methods of preventing its entrance, but shortly had to direct their attention to its cure.

John W. Francis sent a series of letters to James Bond Read, chairman of the Medical Board of Savannah, and later published them in pamphlet form. He distinguished three stages of the disease and prescribed a treatment for each: the first stage was marked by vomiting, diarrhea, heat and thirst; the second showed these conditions aggravated, also visceral congestion and a slowing down of the intellectual faculties and circulation; the last stage found the patient collapsed. His treatment of the first stage was "attention to the primae viae, relieving the bowels of their wonted crudities, and adjusting the common functions of the system;" castor oil, repeated if necessary, rhubarb, magnesia and mint water or a dose of calomel with a few grains of aloes or julap with cream of tartar sufficed. In the second stage he had recourse to bleeding, calomel combined, occasionally, with small doses of opium, blisters to the stomach or poultices to the epigastric region, enemas, and use of frictions in order to restore circulation. In the last stage when there was slight chance of a cure, he suggested bleeding after friction or hot baths to bring the blood to the surface. Likewise for the same purpose, he gave the prescriptions for two liniments commonly used.[54]

In his journal, Graham, who advocated the vegetable diet, records a common preventive policy. He stated that people during the epidemic of 1832 had lived on a "diet of flesh

[54] Francis, John W., *Letters on the Cholera Asphyxia* ... (New York, 1832), *passim*.

and flesh soups, with brandy, port wine and porter."[55] Evidently a common cure, at least in the South, was a combination of opium and camphor, for in 1834 Dr. R. D. Arnold wrote Thomas Spalding that he had not used either of these drugs in treating the slaves belonging to Spalding's son.[56] G. B. Wood proposed the following order of treatment: first, clean out the stomach; second, check the irritation by opium; third, clean the liver by calomel; fourth, place a poultice of mustard over the pit of the stomach; fifth, give one-sixth grain of calomel and one-sixth grain of opium every half hour; and, prescribe a mucilagenous diet for the evacuation of acrid bile.[57] In Cholera Infantum the cure was similar to that recommended for Cholera Asiatic. Rush evacuated the stomach, gave laudanum, teas and cold water, applied plasters, administered tonics and cordials, and sent his patients to convalesce in the country.[58]

While the medical profession could openly war upon most common diseases and prepare for epidemics, its attacks upon venereal diseases were handicapped by the common prejudice of the people, even of the profession. The consensus of opinion was that these diseases were divine punishment for licentious living and as such should be left to run their course. Consequently little was known of them and their cure. Sydenham in the seventeenth century considered gonorrhea and syphilis as the same disease,[59] and Thomas, as late as 1811, subscribed to this error.[60] Even in 1826, a writer in

[55] *The Graham Journal of Health and Longevity* (Boston, 1837-1839), I, p. 178.

[56] Arnold, Richard D., *Letters of ... 1808-1876*, Ed. R. H. Shryock (Duke University Papers of the Trinity College Historical Society. Double Series, XVIII-XIX), p. 12.

[57] Wood, *op. cit.*, I, p. 650.

[58] Rush, *op. cit.*, I, pp. 160 *et seq.*

[59] Sydenham, *op. cit.*, II, p. 17.

[60] Thomas, *op. cit.*, p. 440.

the *New England Journal of Medicine and Surgery* stated, " It will be perceived, that I have noticed gonorrhœa as one of the primary forms of syphilis. I am aware that a majority of enlightened practitioners consider gonorrhoea and chancre as distinct diseases." [61]

With this general attitude towards social diseases, it is not surprising that they should have been comparatively neglected. Gregory, after failing with sarsaparilla, nitric acid, opium and guiacum, found mercury useful, particularly in the cure of syphilis. When discharge stopped, gonorrhea patients were optimistically declared well. Other cures, such as cubebs, were in vogue in the third decade of the nineteenth century.[62] The *Medical Intelligencer* said,

A dessertspoonful of powdered Cubebs, taken six times daily in water, is useful in early acute clap. Unless relief follows in 6 days, cubebs should be discontinued. If its use be interrupted on first appearance of cure relapse follows. Its medicinal property, probably resides in its volatile oil.[63]

The same journal quoted the London *Lancet*, in which a sailor said that a mixture of powdered black pepper and gin had cured many a sailor lad.[64] Nitric acid and nitrate of silver complete the list of common remedies for gonorrhea.[65] It is obvious from this brief survey of venereal disease that nature did most of the mending. Doctors seem to have considered the diseases rather lightly, especially gonorrhea, and after superficial treatment they discharged the " clap " patient.

[61] *New England Journal of Medicine and Surgery*, XV, p. 159.

[62] *Philadelphia Journal of Medical and Physical Sciences* (9 volumes, 1820-1824; n. s. 5 volumes, 1825-1827, Phila., 1820-1827), IV, p. 314.

[63] *Boston Medical Intelligencer*, I, pp. 383-389.

[64] *Ibid.*, IV, p. 23.

[65] *American Journal of Medical Sciences*, XX, p. 10 contains account of nitrate of silver, and many articles appeared on the question of nitric acid.

THE TREATMENT OF INSANITY

Prior to the work of Philip Pinel, whose efforts with the insane at the time of the French Revolution have centered attention upon him as the pioneer in humane treatment, the care of the insane is one of the saddest chapters in history. Treatment of the mentally unfit in America during the years from the Revolution to 1850 may be separated into three stages. In the first, the insane and feeble-minded were outside the pale of medical attention. As social and family disgraces, incapable of improvement, they were chained, imprisoned or otherwise rendered harmless; or, if they seemed peaceful, they were left at large. In the second stage, they were committed to hospitals where various efforts were made to cure them; or they were treated according to common practice by local physicians. In the last stage, asylums were established with emphasis upon "moral treatment," which consisted of kindliness and sympathy in order to arouse the patient's mind. These three stages coexisted in the United States. While some lunatics were living in unspeakable conditions in the county jails, others were receiving attention from experienced physicians in clean and healthful asylums. At the same time, other asylums were conducted on old-fashioned principles, and the inmates suffered a medication hardly less terrorizing than chains.

Committing insane to jails and almshouses resulted from the belief in their incurability and their insensibility to cold and other pain.[66] Cold has the additional value of numbing the maniac into harmlessness. When patients were violent, they were chained or manacled; thus a man in Massachusetts was tied by the ankles and subjected to freezing weather for

---

[66] New York State. *Senate Document No. 20, New York State Asylum Report, 1838-1842* (Albany, 1842), pp. 5-6.

twenty years.[67] Dorothea Dix pictures conditions in the Albany County Alms-House in 1844:

> Ascending a flight of stairs, conducting from without, to the second story of a large building, I entered an apartment not clean, not ventilated, and over-heated; here were several females chiefly in the state of dementia; they were decently dressed but otherwise exhibited personal neglect; the beds were sufficiently comfortable; the hot air, foul and noisome vapors, produced a sense of suffocation impossible to be long endured.

She then forced an entrance into the men's department, located in the cellar, where she found nakedness and cold as the methods of quieting the inmates.[68]

Beginning with the Pennsylvania Hospital in 1751 various general hospitals were organized with insane departments; among them were the New York Hospital, The Charity Hospital of New Orleans and the Massachusetts General Hospital. The first hospital exclusively for the insane was founded by Virginia in 1769 and occupied in 1773.[69] Although these asylums did not introduce the new moral treatment, their staffs did accept the theory brilliantly defended at a later date by Benjamin Rush, that insanity was a disease subject to medical treatment. In 1786 Rush, in an address entitled "An Inquiry into the Influence of Physical Causes upon the Moral Faculty", pointed out the intimate connection between the activity of the mind and the condition of the body. He stated that "our books of medicine contain many records of the effects of physical causes upon the memory, the imagi-

---

[67] Waterson, R. C., *The Condition of the Insane in Massachusetts* (Boston, 1843), pp. 1-2.

[68] Dix, D. L., *Memorial* [soliciting enlarged and improved accommodations for the insane of the State of New York] (Albany, 1844), pp. 6-7. Her petitions give a clear picture of conditions throughout the country.

[69] New York Academy of Medicine. *Transactions* (New York, 1847), I, pp. 2-31.

nation, and the judgment " and that cases wherein demented people had been cured justified medical treatment. Throughout the address he stressed the interplay of mind and body; in fact, much of his address seems strangely like behaviorism.[70] Methods of treatment in 1790 have been described as follows:

Then came a change for the better though accompanied by Dr. Rush's profuse bleeding and the aid of cold water, chains, and the whip, all of which seem to have been in use in the first American Asylum for the insane, [A branch of the Pennsylvania Hospital and therefore not exclusively devoted to mental cases] opened at Philadelphia, under Dr. Franklin's eye, in 1752.[71]

The conditions in the early asylums aroused public fear and distrust; hence as late as 1843 the Eastern Asylum of Virginia attempted to dissipate false impressions by stating that " the old gratings, with their prison-like appearance and partial insecurity, have been replaced by the neatness and security of modern castings." [72]

Gradually new methods of caring for the insane developed in France and England. The authorities attempted to arouse the patient's interest, avoided the use of cold baths and bleeding and provided about one attendant to every ten patients instead of one to every thirty or sixty.[73] Beginning with the Friends Retreat at Frankford, Pennsylvania, in 1817, the asylums were built and organized on these principles. In chronological order they were the McLean, a

[70] Tuke, D. H., *The Insane of the United States and Canada* (London, 1885), p. 7; Rush, Benj., *An Inquiry in to the Influence of Physical Causes upon the Moral Faculty* (Phila., 1839), *passim*.

[71] Sanborn, F. D., Ed. *Memoir of Pliny Earle, M. D....* (Boston, 1898), p. viii.

[72] Virginia, Eastern Lunatic Asylum. *Report for 1843* (Richmond, 1844), p. 42.

[73] New York State. *Senate Document, No. 20*, pp. 5-6.

branch of the Massachusetts General Hospital in 1818 and the Bloomingdale Hospital, a branch of the New York Hospital. South Carolina built its asylum in 1822, Connecticut founded the Hartford Retreat in 1823, Kentucky established a hospital at Lexington the following year and Virginia built one at Staunton in 1828. During the next ten years Massachusetts founded a state institution at Worcester (1833); the Pennsylvania Hospital erected its building at Mantua (beginning it in 1832 and completing it in 1839); Maryland established an asylum in Baltimore in 1834; Vermont began construction in Brattleboro in 1837; New York City cared for its insane on Blackwell's Island in 1838; Boston, Tennessee and Ohio built hospitals in the next year. Maine, New Hampshire and New York (Utica) built retreats in 1840, 1842 and 1843. Indiana fell into line in 1848. In the following two years Illinois completed its building in 1849 and Louisiana in 1850. From 1848 to 1850, North Carolina, Mississippi and Michigan made plans to house their mental defectives.[74] It is significant that these institutions were, with the exception of the McLean, Friends, Pennsylvania and Bloomingdale Hospitals, projects of the states rather than of private philanthropy. As a matter of fact the states were very generous; for example, New York, by 1839, had spent $431,636 on its state hospital at Utica and, the Worcester Asylum in Massachusetts privately endowed to some extent but largely state-supported, was spending nearly $50,000 yearly by 1850.[75]

[74] Dix, D. L., *Memorial ... for the Relief and Support of the Indigent Curable and Incurable Insane in the United States* (Washington, 1848), pp. 6-7; New York State. *Senate Document No. 20*, pp. 60-61. Lists private asylums; *Michigan, Laws of ... 1848* (Detroit, 1848), pp. 246-248; *Mississippi, Code of . . . 1798-1848*, pp. 306-307; *North Carolina, Acts of ... 1848-1849* (Raleigh, 1849), pp. 3-13.

[75] New York State. *Senate Document No. 20*, 1842, p. 1; State Lunatic Hospital, Worcester, Massachusetts; *Annual Reports 1-18, 1832-1850* (Worcester, 1833-1850), 1850.

At their meeting in Philadelphia in 1851, the superintendents laid down a number of rules for prospective asylums. The buildings should be situated at a minimum distance of two miles from a town; the plot of land should be proportioned at a rate of 100 acres to 250 patients, with fifty acres of gardens and pleasure grounds; it should also be near facilities for 10,000 gallons of water a day. Plans should be approved by a physician. The capacity should not exceed 250 patients, but 200 was preferable. The building should be stone or brick containing eight wards for each sex; the wards required a parlor, corridor, single lodging rooms, dormitory, communicating chambers for two attendants, clothes room, bath room, water closet, dining room, dumb waiter and speaking tube. The rooms, eight by ten by twelve feet as a minimum, should have windows with confining apartments above ground. The floors of the room should be made of wood, but stairways of iron or stone were preferable. The best construction should be a main building for administration with wings containing well-ventilated corridors. Gas was recommended for lighting. An ideal institution would include: an apartment for washing clothes separated from the rest of the building; underground drainage; hot-air heat; forced ventilation; boilers in a separate building; water closets of indestructible material; floors of bath rooms and similar conveniences of non-absorbent material; wards with corridors ten feet wide and large windows for excitable patients; and, finally, the building should be so disguised that the patients would not feel imprisoned. The cost of such a structure including furniture was estimated, in Philadelphia, at $200,000.[76] Most of these features were incorporated in the New Jersey Asylum for the

---

[76] Kirkbride, Thomas, *On the Construction, Organization and General Arrangements of Hospitals for the Insane* (Phila., 1854), App. pp. 76-78, 30.

Insane at Trenton, which became a model for its time, a Massachusetts committee recommending it to the state in 1848.[17]

The institutions were organized under trustees or managers who appointed the treasurer and the superintendent, who was a physician; he in turn selected the matron, often his wife, and the staff. Thomas Kirkbride, of the Pennsylvania asylum at Mantua, set the following salaries as fair compensation for the staff administering to 250 patients: chief physician, $1500 with board and room for himself and family, or $2500 without maintenance; the first assistant physician and steward, $500; the second assistant physician and matron, $300; the supervising female attendant, $175; the male teacher, $200; the female teacher, $150; each of the sixteen male attendants, $168; and each of the sixteen female attendants, $108.[18] Actual salaries did not differ much from this recommendation, for in the report on the New York asylum in 1842 the salaries of many superintendents were stated, ranging from $1000 and maintenance for the superintendent of the Vermont asylum to $1500 and accommodations for the more highly paid men.[19]

Although physicians in 1850 were still unaware of the nature and causes of mental disease, they had made progress in the care of the insane. The division of insanity into monomania, mania, dementia, moral and incoherent insanity continued. With regard to causes the report mentioned many different possibilities. Common causes, listed by superintendents, were intemperance, ill health, masturbation, domestic affliction, religion, property worries, disappointed

[17] Massachusetts. *Insanity, Committee on...: Report of the joint Committee of the Legislature of Massachusetts Appointed April 20, 1848* (Boston, 1849), p. 28.
[18] Kirkbride, *op. cit.*, pp. 32-53.
[19] New York State. *Senate Document No. 20*, pp. 64 *et seq.*

affection and ambition, epilepsy, puerperal fever, wounds and abuses of snuff.[80] Thomas Kirkbride, an eminent superintendent of his time, said in his report for 1841, " We have not placed *hereditary predisposition* among the causes in this table—for without something special to induce the attack, an individual thus disposed, who leads a proper course of life, has good reason to expect immunity from the disease." [81] Samuel Woodward of Worcester said that the truth lay between those who denied hereditary predisposition and those who regarded it as the sole cause of insanity.[82] Although Pliny Earle, Superintendent of Bloomingdale, first described in 1847 a case of paresis, syphilis received no attention as a factor in mental diseases.[83] The commonly listed causes, however, were those reported by friends or relatives responsible for the inmates.

Before discussing the attempts to cure insanity through hospitalization it is well to state the treatment commonly used by the general practitioner. Prevailing medication has been accurately described in verse form, by Samuel Thomson, whose satirical jibes at the medical profession were not without influence.

Recipe To Cure a Crazy Man

Soon as the man is growing mad,
Send for a doctor, have him bled:
Take from his arm two quarts at least,
Nearly as much as kills a beast.

---

[80] State Lunatic Hospital, Worcester, Massachusetts. *Report, 1841*, p. 40.

[81] Pennsylvania Hospital for the Insane. *Reports, 1841-1846* (Phila., 1846), p. 40.

[82] New York State. *Senate Document No. 20*, p. 105.

[83] Sanborn, *op. cit.*, p. 161.

But if bad symptoms yet remain,
He must tap another vein;
Soon as the doctor has him bled;
Then draw a blister on his head.

Next he comes, as it is said,
The blistered skin takes from his head;
The laud'num gives to ease his pain,
Till he can visit him again.

The doctor says he's so insane,
It must be dropsy on the brain,
To lay the heat while yet in bed,
A cap of ice lays on his head.

And lest the fever should take hold,
The nitre gives to keep him cold;
And if distraction should remain,
He surely must be bled again.

The bowels now have silent grown,
The *choledocus* lost its tone;
He then, bad humours to expel,
The jalap gives with calomel.

The physic works, you well must know,
Till he can neither stand nor go;
If any heat should still remain,
The lancet must be used again.

The man begins to pant for breath,
The doctor says he's struck with death;
All healing medicine is denied,
I fear the man is mortified.

. . . .

What sickness, sorrow, pain, and wo,
The human race do undergo,
By learned quacks, who sickness make,
I fear, for filthy lucre's sake.[84]

[84] Thomson, Samuel, *Learned Quackery Exposed*... (Boston, 1836), pp. 8-9.

The great contribution to the care of the insane, then, was the gradual abandonment of such methods. Moral treatment became common practice. Buildings were set in pleasant surroundings. As far as possible, prison-like features were eliminated, and demented persons were treated with consideration and sympathy. Attendants were particularly important in such treatment. The rules of the New Jersey Asylum at Trenton are typical. Attendants were required to show the patients respect and good will, to oversee their cleanliness and dress and to supervise them in their bedmaking and similar activities. They were particularly forbidden to lay hands on a patient without permission of the superintendent unless the patient were harming himself. They had to guard the inmates at meals, to prevent them from obtaining knives or other dangerous implements, to prevent outside communication, to watch suicidal patients at night and to give the patients their medicine.[85]

In addition most asylums either abolished or limited the use of restraining apparatus. The Maryland Hospital for the Insane stated that:

With respect to corporal restraints, we have to say, that we are not yet prepared to give them up entirely; the mildest forms only are used, but never unless directed by the physician. With us they are never resorted to as punishment, but merely as a necessary means to prevent the patient doing mischief; and of this we endeavor to make him sensible.[86]

Ohio restricted such apparatus to quarrelsome people who were restrained by leathern wristbands, to destructive or suicidal persons who wore mittens, and to violent persons who

[85] New Jersey State Lunatic Asylum at Trenton. *By-Laws, Adopted by the Managers of ... 1847* (Trenton, 1848), pp. 16-19.

[86] Maryland Hospital for the Insane. *Reports, 1844-1850* (with the exception of 1845) (Baltimore, 1845-1852), 1844, p. 11.

were secluded. This hospital, also, used cold and warm baths and relied upon the word of honor of the patients.[87] The reports do not indicate whether such a disciplinary code was successful.

Moral treatment included the substitution of kindliness and sympathy for restricting apparatus in the hospitals, and the attempt to restore the patient by pleasant work which would keep him happy. His life in the asylum was designed to awaken his consciousness and to restore him to sanity by a regime which would build him up physically. The Pennsylvania Hospital listed in 1841 the activities in which patients engaged as outdoor labor, workshops, cleaning the house, reading in a library of nine hundred volumes, sewing, walking, riding in the carriage, and playing such games as chess.[88] By 1846 this hospital and Bloomingdale had established complete courses of popular lectures for the patients.[89] An inmate of the Maryland Hospital could read such authors as Gibbon, Hume, Smollett and Goldsmith.[90] Finally, religious worship was permitted on Sunday.[91]

The purpose, then, behind moral treatment was to give patients occpations which they liked. No force was brought to bear, but they were encouraged to work in the fields or, in the case of women, to sew and to do household tasks. Together with this treatment, the profession continued to use with decreasing emphasis a course of medication. Amariah Brigham, Superintendent of the Utica Asylum, stated that there was no specific remedy for insanity. When the mental

---

[87] Ohio Lunatic Asylum, Columbus. *Annual Report* (1839-1845, Columbus, 1840-1846), 1841-1842, pp. 67-70.

[88] Pennsylvania Hospital for the Insane. *Report*, 1841, pp. 25-33.

[89] *Ibid.*, 1846, pp. 20-21; Earle, Pliny, *Bloomingdale*... (N. Y., 1848), p. 35; State Hospital, Worcester, Massachusetts. *Report*, 1843, pp. 79-81.

[90] Maryland Hospital for the Insane. *Report*, 1844, p. 9.

[91] Worcester, *Report*, 1836, pp. 29-30.

disorder was of recent origin he preferred the antiphlogistic course (bloodletting), but in cases of prolonged grief, ill-health and similar circumstances he recommended tonics or opiates. Although he condemned Rush for overuse of bleeding, he constantly resorted to the procedure himself. Whenever mental derangement had been caused by a blow on the head, he prescribed cathartics; and for the patient who was suffering from nervous excitement, he regarded topical bleeding, warm or cold water to the head and laxatives as a successful treatment. He found that "pouring cold water, in a small stream from a height of four or five feet directly upon the head, is generally one of the most certain means of subduing violent maniacal excitement we have ever seen tried," but he admonished that it be done gently! Warm baths and croton oil subdued violent patients. On the other hand, he had little faith in blisters, issues or setons in the neck. Laudanum was sometimes employed to quiet patients. After making suggestions in specific cases, he advised physicians to search for other diseases as the cause of insanity and to use cod-liver oil to build up vitality.[92] Defective as this system was, it was a decided improvement over head-shaving, blistering, and scalp bleeding which were in vogue, as late as 1840, in so humane an asylum as that run by the Society of Friends at Frankford, Pennsylvania.[93]

The asylums accommodated as many patients as possible, but a large number remained outside their doors either as incurables or unfortunate individuals for whom no room existed. There were in the United States in 1840 some 17,434 insane persons.[94] By 1848 when Dorothea Dix petitioned Congress to aid asylums, not over 3000 of the insane could be

[92] New York State Asylum, Utica. *Report* (Utica, 1849), pp. 47-55.
[93] Sanborn, *op. cit.*, p. 155.
[94] Ohio Asylum for the Insane, Columbus. *Report*, 1840-1841, p. 31.

housed in the existing institutions.[95] If the asylums' claim of cures, running as high as ninety percent, had been valid, the so-called recent cases of insanity could have been rapidly returned to public life. The apparent effectiveness of these cures, no doubt, lay in the practice of taking only recent cases and ignoring the patients who returned subsequently to undergo further treatment.

We have now surveyed the asylums for the insane which developed in the United States from 1783 to 1850. Although there were more spectacular achievements in the fields of surgery and midwifery, none was more thorough and indicative of future change in medicine than the removal of thousands of outcasts from their jails, dungeons and outbuildings, where they were beaten or frozen into submission, to hospitals, where they were well-fed and treated by methods designed to improve their lot. Many factors enter into this change. First is the inevitable recoil from the revelation of the conditions which existed at the time Pinel made his famous excursion into the cells where the insane of Paris were imprisoned. Furthermore, the treatment of the insane in the early years of this period was based upon the age-old conviction that they could not be helped. When it was discovered that their condition could be improved, and their malady at times completely cured, the work of investigation into methods of treatment gained momentum. And the insane were among the numerous unfortunates who profited from the general humanitarianism which was a nineteenth-century manifestation of the philosophy of human perfectibility so deeply cherished by the champions of the rights of man. In a society which was convinced of its rapid progress toward the millennium it is not strange to find philanthropic persons who made the plight of the insane their lively concern.

[95] Dix, D. L., *Memorial . . . for the Relief and Support of the Indigent Curable and Incurable Insane in the United States*, pp. 6-7.

At the head of these benevolent persons one may place Benjamin Rush. Samuel B. Woodward, superintendent of McLean, credited Rush with anticipating Philip Pinel in his address " An Essay on the Influence of Physical Causes upon the Moral Faculty," delivered to the American Philosophical Society in 1786.[96] We have already seen how Rush explained insanity as a disease subject to medication. He felt that the moral lapses were explainable by the mental condition. Naturally, hospitals had been established before this address, but he brought to public attention (the legislature of Pennsylvania was present) the curability of the insane.

A more influential character was Dorothea Dix. Born in Maine, April 4, 1802, she entered upon her active life in Massachusetts, where she established a school in Worcester at the age of fifteen. Later she taught in Boston, but her marriage interrupted her activities. Finally, in 1841, aroused by stories of the plight of the feeble-minded, she turned her attention to their needs. Gradually she entered upon the work which was to take her up and down the land. Boldly, in a generation which believed that a woman belonged in the home, she examined conditions in the states and petitioned the various state legislatures for asylums or reform of existing institutions. Her facts were collected in personal investigations, and they were presented without a qualm. The extent of her travels can be obtained from a list of her petitions. In 1844, she petitioned the New York legislature; in 1845 that of Pennsylvania; in 1846, that of Kentucky; in 1848, Congress; in 1847, Tennessee; in 1849, Alabama; and in 1850, Mississippi. When one considers that she prefaced these petitions, which were often personally presented, with investigation, the amount of labor and time seem prodigious. The results of her efforts can be traced in the building of hospitals during these years and in the

[96] Worcester, *Report*, 1841, pp. 69-70.

districts which she canvassed. Obviously one cannot give Mrs. Dix sole credit for these constructions, but her unflagging spirit, and her boldness, which seemed shocking to a generation whose ideas of a woman's conduct were derived from the books of William A. Alcott, often gave new impetus to the efforts being made for the insane. After years of toil she finally broke, physically though not mentally, under the strain and spent her last years as the guest of the New Jersey Asylum at Trenton, in which she died July 17, 1887.[97]

Besides these pioneers, there were exceptional men among the physicians who supervised the asylums. We have already mentioned such theorists as Amariah Brigham, Samuel Woodward and Thomas Kirkbride. Others were Isaac Ray, who supervised the Butler Asylum in Rhode Island and whose book on insanity was a noteworthy contribution to medical jurisprudence, William A. Awl of the Ohio Asylum, Pliny Earle, who did so much at Bloomingdale, and among early physicians, Rufus Wyman of McLean. These men and other superintendents came together in the Society of Medical Superintendents and Physicians of Hospitals and Asylums for the Insane in the United States at a meeting in Philadelphia in 1844, and thenceforth cooperated to better conditions.[98] Their work, however, was furthered by the medical societies. In Connecticut, Alabama, New Jersey and Ohio this aid was gratefully acknowledged by the superintendents.

MIDWIFERY

An increasing interest in obstetrics, which removed many cases from the hands of midwives to those of regular physicians, characterized this period. As a result of the earlier

[97] Tiffany, Francis, *Life of Dorothea Lynde Dix* (Boston, 1890), *passim*.

[98] *American Journal of Insanity* (Volumes I-VI, Utica, 1844-1850), I, 1844.

work of Shippen, and especially after Valentine Seaman's course for midwives in 1798 in New York, the medical colleges created professorships to promote the study of midwifery. Despite the fact that women had handled most cases, some doctors had taken enough interest to perfect instruments and to write aphorisms on the subject.

Many reasons may be advanced for this ignorance which was greater, probably, than in other fields of medicine. Of especial significance was early Christian tradition which regarded childbearing as a part of the curse upon Eve. When suffering is accepted as inevitable by people, efforts are not made to overcome it. The Protestant Revolt had not materially modified this phase of Christian tradition, and it remained for the generations after 1800 to apply their energy, in many cases against the wishes of the clergy, to ameliorate woman's position. The other factor, which is closely related to the attitude of earlier Christianity, was the excessive modesty of women. In comparison with the old practice of delivery performed by a doctor who could not even see the external organs, some progress was possible in dealing with modest women who objected only to internal examinations. R. Lee's statement that many would not permit an internal examination in cases of miscarriage illustrates the difficulties of the obstetrician.[99] Writing in 1838 to Dr. Charles D. Meigs of Philadelphia, Dr. Arnold of Savannah, explained the attitude of his own wife:

As the wife of a medical man, she is aware that false delicacy too often injures females, by their allowing disease to get beyond the reach of medical art before they speak out. I have told her to answer any questions you should think necessary to ask her.[100]

[99] Lee, R., *Lectures on the Theory and Practice of Midwifery* ... (Phila., 1844), p. 192.
[100] Arnold, *op. cit.*, p. 18.

THE PRACTICE OF PHYSICK

Despite obvious handicaps, the medical profession did concern itself with the causes of generation. Experimentation being out of the question, speculation stressed three theories. These were: (1) the child is a mixture of the molecules of the father and the mother; (2) the child, fully developed in microscopic dimensions, comes wholly from the father, the term animalcule being applied to the microscopic child; and (3) the child comes wholly from the egg of the mother. Charles D. Meigs, a recognized authority on midwifery, confessed his own ignorance of the subject.[101] Without knowledge of the origin of the child, the profession had difficulty in explaining or curing sterility. As early as 1810 cold baths, chalybeate medicines, separation from the husband in cases of profuse menses, and, when corpulence in the woman was considered the cause, moderate exercise and nitrous acid were advised.[102] Although men were considered the source in the animalcules theory, the profession did not blame them for sterility. Oxygen, like most new discoveries, received consideration in the theory ascribing sterility to the absence of that element at the time of conception. In substantiation of this theory, an article in the *Medical Repository,* pointed to the " astonishing number of births among the negroes " who were less private in their habits and consequently had the advantage of fresh air.[103]

Professional willingness to utilize new drugs evidenced itself in the increased use of ergot. Frenchmen had long observed that ergot, a rust which appears upon rye, was chewed by cows to ease calving; midwives in European

---

[101] Meigs, C. D., *The Philadelphia Practice of Midwifery* (Phila., 1838), pp. 85-100.

[102] Burns, T., *The Principles of Midwifery Including the Diseases of Women and Children*, with notes by N. Chapman (Phila., 1810), pp. 124-125.

[103] *Medical Repository*, X, p. 131.

countries had long been aware of its value.[104] Although Haggard attributes its introduction into America to Stevens and Hosack of New York City,[105] a writer in the *New England Journal of Medicine and Surgery* in 1818 said that it had been introduced in 1809 by Dr. John Stearns, then of Albany, who received it from Lyman Spalding.[106] However that may be, ergot was brought to America in the early nineteenth century and, after much criticism and discussion in the medical journals, was approved by the profession. Prophetic of its course is a statement by Dr. A. W. Ives in the *Medical Repository* for 1820:

Such will ever be the infatuation, on the introduction of a new and potent medicine. Before its virtues can accurately be ascertained, and precisely estimated, it must be subjected to inordinate and indiscreet use; and as in some diseases it will prove injurious, and under some circumstances appear inert, it will generally be discarded for a while (after having been too highly extolled) as a remedy of hazardous operation or of doubtful efficacy.[107]

For the guidance of midwives and physicians elaborate directions were frequently published. According to a procedure recommended in 1844, the patient was prepared for delivery by the substitution of a "shift" or nightgown for other clothing. To set up the delivery bed a mattress was placed over a feather bed, a sheep-skin or water-proof cloth over the mattress and finally a blanket over the sheep-skin. The expectant mother was placed so that she could brace her feet against the left side of the bed while grasping a towel tied to the right bed post.[108] The room was kept cool, and a few

[104] Haggard, H. W., *op. cit.*, pp. 218-219.
[105] *Ibid.*, p. 219.
[106] *New England Journal of Medicine and Surgery*, VII, p. 146.
[107] *Medical Repository*, XXI, p. 20.
[108] Lee, *op. cit.*, pp. 224-225.

THE PRACTICE OF PHYSICK 133

people were allowed around the bed. Since the doctor was in attendance during this period, he might give tea or coffee with dry toast to a hungry patient.[109]

With the completion of these preparations, the patient was examined. As long as this examination was limited to questions modesty was not outraged, but an internal examination had to be suggested with tact. It was generally agreed, especially in the case of the first child, that the best approach to a woman was by way of the nurse. Permission granted, the examination proceeded without regard to hygiene by placing the patient in a horizontal position and using the forefinger, lubricated by cold cream, lard or soap, as the instrument.

If the birth was normal, child and mother received little medical assistance. Although in cases of weakness a small quantity of wine was permissible, the early practice of such stimulants as cordials gave way, shortly after 1800, to tea and gruel. While the physician guarded against fatigue, he permitted the patient to walk around the room.[110] If necessary, the bowels were kept open by castor oil.[111] In normal births with the exception of protecting the perineum and preventing too rapid birth little was done; in difficult births, the head might be moved slowly from side to side in order to loosen the body.[112] When the face of the child appeared, it was washed; and when the child was expelled, the umbilical cord was tied. While turning the placenta around several times to prevent attachment to the membranes, tight bandages or " napkins " were applied to the abdomen; these were gradually tightened, and the placenta removed by pulling on

[109] Burns, *op. cit.*, 194-195.
[110] *Ibid.*, pp. 195-196.
[111] Rigby, E., *A System of Midwifery* (Phila., 1841), p. 104.
[112] Smellie, William, *A Treatise on the Theory and Practice of Midwifery* (2 volumes, London, 1779), I, p. 185.

the umbilical cord. Delivery completed, the patient was washed and " put to bed ", which consisted of changing her nightgown and shifting her to the other side of the bed. The doctor remained an hour to guard against hemorrhage, gave an opiate, and prescribed gruel tea or barley water for forty-eight to sixty hours.[113] Rigby, writing in 1841, advised applying the child to the breast soon after its birth instead of waiting three days, the previous practice of the profession.[114]

Practice in abnormal births was largely individualistic. Doctors relied upon two instruments, the forceps and the vectis, the latter instrument resembling one blade of the forceps with half of its thirteen inches consisting of a wooden handle. Improvements in these instruments were slight, the forceps, which had been invented by Chamberlen in the seventeenth century, remaining practically unchanged. Forceps, which Lee felt had been over-used in the first forty years of the nineteenth century, were utilized in protracted labor or in feeble action but not in cases of difficult labor.[116] After the head had rested six hours, forceps might be inserted, first the right blade and then the left, over the ears, locked and operation begun. While moving the child, particular care was required.[117] Although its use to correct malposition in the pelvic cavity was condemned, the vectis functioned as a lever to aid normal action.[118] If birth was impossible or

[113] Dewees, W. P., *A Compendious System of Midwifery* (Phila., 1824), pp. 199-200; Lee, *op. cit.*, pp. 225-229.

[114] Rigby, *op. cit.*, p. 118.

[115] Lee, *op. cit.*, pp. 290-291; the modifications in the instrument were made by Smellie and Denman, p. 294.

[116] *Ibid.*, pp. 11 and 301.

[117] Denman, T., *Aphorisms on the Application and use of the Forceps and Vectis...* (Phila., 1803), pp. 14-15, 17-20, 21-23.

[118] Churchill, F., *On the Theory and Practice of Midwifery.* With notes and additions by Robert M. Huston (Phila., 1843), p. 97.

the child died, the doctor reduced the size of the head by perforation which released the brain. Then the child was removed by hooking the fingers in the head cavity.[119] Despite the fact that he had never seen a cæsarian section, Lee advised it in cases when normal birth seemed impossible.[120] Rigby gave opium to ease the pain during such an operation.[121]

In abortion, bloodletting, opium and light diet was recommended, while in case of hemorrhage an astringent or ergot in conjunction with cold applications was common practice. To prevent regular abortion a hard mattress and cool room were ordered.[122] Lee, in a detailed discussion, stated that when the orifice of the uterus was closed the methods to stop hemorrhage and uterine contraction were the following: bleeding at the arm with the body in a horizontal position; ice in a bladder, or a napkin soaked with vinegar, or water applied to the upper stomach; a light diet and cold drinks; two grains of superacetate of lead and one-fourth grain of opium every three hours, or the infusion of roses with dilute sulphuric acid and a few drops of an opiate at intervals. After several weeks of this treatment, he advised a better diet and gentle exercise in the fresh air. In case the abortion became more serious, he hastened action by ergot in scruple doses. If this failed, he removed the fetus, using the fore and middle fingers as a forceps, since "they are the only forceps that can be used for this purpose."[123]

[119] Rigby, *op. cit.*, pp. 161-164.

[120] Lee, *op. cit.*, p. 320; the first such case was performed in America in 1794 by Jesse Bennett, a Virginia physician. Fielding H. Garrison in the Mayo Lectures: *Contributions of the West to American Medicine* (Phila. and London, 1933), p. 166.

[121] Rigby, *op. cit.*, p. 156.

[122] Tucker, D. H., *Elements of the Principles and Practice of Midwifery* (Phila., 1848), pp. 309-401.

[123] Lee, *op. cit.*, pp. 192-193.

If the mother survived a normal or abnormal delivery, she always faced that horror of an unsanitary age, puerperal fever. The remedies for ordinary convulsions—bleeding, emetics, clysters and opiates,[124] and other medications, such as castor oil, opium, morphine, poultices of linseed meal and warm poultices, were rarely efficacious in the treatment of puerperal fever. Foxglove, late in the period, was used with some success.[125] The medical profession was slow to recognize the contagious nature of puerperal fever. When Oliver Wendell Holmes presented this idea to the Boston Society for Medical Improvement in 1843, he failed to substantiate his theory by statistics.[126] Until sometime after the experiments by Semmelweiss, the famous Hungarian practitioner, in Vienna in 1847 established the truth of Holmes's contention, American physicians approved the attitude of Charles D. Meigs, a leading authority in Philadelphia, who stated that mortality in puerperal fever was the "justification of Providence, a judgment instituted to remind us of the sin committed by the mother of the race." [127]

Since the great majority of births were normal, attention centered upon the child as soon as it was born. Numerous were the methods used to induce breathing. In the first five minutes the application of the mouth was tried. If that failed a small bellows was applied to each nostril in turn, the other nostril being kept closed. In some cases the chest was alternately pressed and released. If the infant failed to respond to these treatments, it was then immersed in a warm bath of ninety-six degrees temperature. Occasionally

[124] Denman, *Aphorisms*, p. 106.

[125] Blundell, J., *Lectures on the Principles and Practice of Midwifery* (Phila., 1842), p. 459; Rigby, *op. cit.*, p. 274; Lee, *op. cit.*, pp. 504-506.

[126] Holmes, Oliver W., *Medical Essays* (Boston, 1911), p. 105.

[127] Atkinson, Donald T., *Life Sketches of Great Physicians* (N. Y., 1922), p. 134.

THE PRACTICE OF PHYSICK

physicians tried snuff or ammonia as a stimulant, or resorted to the practice of bleeding at the umbilical cord before ligating it.[128] Dewees placed the child face downward, the head lower than the hips and then gently shook it in order to release the mucus.[129]

After these preliminaries, the normal child received a teaspoonful of castor oil, was placed in a well-aired room and was given a diet of mother's milk.[130] Regularity of feedings was considered important by Gooch, who, while suggesting a wet nurse under thirty, preferred the milk of a domesticated animal, such as a goat.[131] Three days after delivery a mild laxative was given to the mother. Her diet during lactation consisted, in the first few days, of gruel tapioca, arrowroot and other light foods and thereafter eggs, chicken and similar foods until stronger meats were given.[132] If the mother did not nurse the child, the breasts were reduced by lightly-covered shoulders, cold applications, laxatives and a light diet. Rigby stated that nursing prevented pregnancy during a period as high as twenty-four months but usually only for twelve months.[133] According to Dr. Copeland of Boston the proper time to wean a child was between eighteen months and two years.[134] If desired, vaccination took place the first and third month;[135] other operations, such as that for ruptured umbilicus, took place two weeks or more after birth and that for harelip at the end of three months.[136]

[128] Gooch, R., *A Practical Compendium of Midwifery*... (Phila., 1832), pp. 278-280.
[129] Dewees, *Midwifery*, p. 195.
[130] Gooch, *op. cit.*, p. 277.
[131] Lee, *op. cit.*, p. 230.
[132] Rigby, *op. cit.*, p. 121.
[133] *Ibid.*, p. 122.
[134] *Boston Medical Intelligencer*, IV, p. 475.
[135] Gooch, *op. cit.*, pp. 278-280.
[136] *Ibid.*, pp. 281-286.

SURGERY

During periods of our survey the discovery of the anesthetic use of ether was the most sensational contribution to surgery. Although this discovery stands out brilliantly against a drab medical background, it is important to remember that it came at the end and not at the beginning of the period. For years the ordinary practitioner, who depended partly upon the crops of his field for an income, attempted to remove foreign bodies or to amputate limbs with instruments of doubtful merit and based his incisions upon a scanty knowledge of anatomy. He labored under two difficulties: operating upon a conscious patient; and operating without an understanding of aseptic surgery.

True as these statements are, there was real progress in the use of instruments and in the dexterity with which unusual operations were performed. Among the more famous operations were Ephraim McDowell's ovariotomy in 1809 and Marion Simms's operation for vesico-vaginal fistula in 1849.[137] Probably the most dexterous surgeon of this period was Valentine Mott. Son of a Quaker doctor, he was born August 20, 1785. In America, he studied under Valentine Seaman and the medical faculty of Columbia College, receiving his medical degree in 1807. In London and Edinburgh, thereafter, he had the advantages of work under Sir Astley Cooper, a famous English surgeon, and James Gregory and Alexander Munro. After his return to America, he became a member of the faculty of Columbia Medical School and later of the College of Physicians and Surgeons. Although he joined the Rutgers Medical School during the quarrel of 1825 and 1826, he returned to the College of Physicians and Surgeons. His further teaching was in the Medical Department of the University of the City of New York.

[137] Garrison in Mayo Lectures, *op. cit.*, pp. 165 and 169.

During these years, he made trips to Europe, partly because of ill-health, and thereby kept up his connection with European surgery. He corresponded with Velpeau, the famous French surgeon, and finally edited his work for American students. His fame as a surgeon rests upon his ligatures of various arteries previously untouched. Although they were unsuccessful in effecting permanent cures of his patients, they won him such fame that he was called to operate upon the Sultan of Turkey. In other operations his skill stood him in good stead, and he justly rose to a position of eminence in the American profession. His death in 1868 brought to an end a career full of honor and of service to the people.[138]

Among the instruments and other aids which these surgeons required were "bistouries, scalpels, dissection forceps, tenaculum and small forceps for arteries, well waxed ligatures, curved needles threaded, fine spone, water warm and cold, wine and hartshorn in case of faintness, assistants to hold the patients" and to give cordials and hand the doctor instruments.[139] Another author increased the length of this list by adding couching needles for eye operations, an open end steel to keep the eye open and a sharp two-edged knife to cut the iris, a perforator in order to keep the eye open while healing, a bent probe for a ligature, an iron instrument for tying the tonsils and a grooved forceps.[140]

In cases of amputation a knife thirteen inches long and a saw seventeen inches long were required.[141] For operations upon the brain common instruments were a spiral perforator

[138] Gross, S. D., *Memoir of Valentine Mott, M. D.* (Phila., 1868), *passim*.

[139] Druitt, R., *The Principles and Practice of Modern Surgery.* Notes by J. B. Flint (Phila., 1842), p. 481.

[140] Sharp, Samuel, *A Treatise on the Operation of Surgery* . . . (London, 1782, 10th ed.), pp. 180-181, 193-195, 203-204.

[141] *Ibid.*, p. 242.

and cylindrical saw with a pin to pierce, equipped with a handle resembling spread wings to grip the pin after the saw had penetrated sufficiently, a button to prevent dust getting into the brain while cleaning the wound, and a jagged forceps to remove bits of bone.[142] Instruments for abdominal operations, practically all of which were for the removal of stone, included a small catheter made of silver, a long-handled knife with a straight point, a silver wire to remove blood or matter which clogged the hollow center of the catheter, a " gorget ", which was a grooved steel instrument for penetrating after the wound was opened, but with blunt edges to prevent it from cutting the sides of the wound; several forceps of various sizes for extracting the stone; and, a spoonlike instrument for scraping pieces of stone or whatever else remained.[143]

For abscesses the medical works recommended a director, a straight-edged knife, a crooked needle, a larger needle for tying arteries and sewing deep wounds, a small one for veins and small wounds, and a very small one for sewing the skin.[144] The list of necessary instruments closed with a proble scissors, a crooked knife with a blunt end, three trocars with sharp points to pierce readily for letting water from the abdomen, a perforator of steel with a wooden handle and a silver point and " sounders " of various sizes for searching for stones in the abdomen.[145]

The importance of minimizing pain during operations and preparing the patient for the inevitable shock which such crude methods entailed led to various efforts to quiet the patient. In cases of " full blooded " individuals, bleeding and sedatives were used.[146] Valentine Mott, in his edition of Velpeau's *Surgery*, said that it was absurd to deny the

[142] *Ibid.*, pp. 159-162.
[143] *Ibid.*, pp. 119-122.
[144] *Ibid.*, pp. lii-liii.
[145] *Ibid.*, pp. 33-34, 117-119.
[146] Druitt, *op. cit.*, p. 582.

THE PRACTICE OF PHYSICK 141

patient's suffering, " for we every day see individuals praying in mercy that we would stop, that we would finish, thus imploring and menacing us, and who would not fail to escape if they were not firmly secured." [147] He then listed the methods in use about 1845 to prevent pain: opium, water of night shade, henbane and lettuce, mesmerism (with a note that it has yet to be confirmed); strapping above the point of the operation in order to numb the nerves (of which practice he disapproved); and, noise to divert the patient. To this list he added that in England and in America and even in Germany many practitioners administered large doses of opium, wine and brandy to their patients even on the day of the operation whereas the French bled their patients into acceptance of their fate.[148] He highly approved of keeping the knife at body temperature to lessen pain, but said, " *to avoid pain* in operation is a chimera that we can no longer pursue in our times." [149]

Against this background of surgical operations, we see the importance of the discovery of the anesthetic use of ether. Ether had, of course, been known to medical men for some time, having been recommended for pulmonary irritation and to relieve suffering in colic and other afflictions, as early as 1815.[150] Horace Wells, a dentist in Hartford, who made use of nitrous oxide and some use of ether while working upon his patients, journeyed to Boston to discuss his efforts with the medical profession of that city. Dr. John C. Warren, son of John Warren and nephew of Joseph Warren, attempted to operate upon a patient who was under the influence of ether; the failure, however, of this operation led him

---

[147] Mott, Valentine, ed. of A. A. L. M. Velpeau, *New Elements of Operative Surgery*. Trans. by P. S. Townsend under the supervision of, and with notes and observations by V. Mott (N. Y., 1847), I, p. 20. This is referred to as Mott's *Velpeau*.

[148] *Ibid.*, I, pp. 22-24, 63.   [149] *Ibid.*, I, p. 24.

[150] *On the Progress of Recent Science*, p. 17.

to drop ether as a possibility. Sometime later, Charles T. Jackson, of Boston, suggested ether to a dentist, C. T. G. Morton, as a means of lessening pain. Morton, after using it, in turn approached Warren with the possibilities of using ether in surgery. This time, September 1846, Warren was successful in his operation. Against Warren's wishes and without further experimentation, the results were published in the newspapers and the *Boston Medical and Surgical Journal*.[151]

Previous to Warren's operation, Crawford Long of Georgia had operated as early as 1842 upon a patient who was anesthetized by ether. Since he did not publish, until 1849, an account of this operation for a tumor upon the neck, he did not receive recognition for his part in the discovery. Charles T. Jackson, who received the Paris medal in 1849 for his part in the introduction of ether as an anesthetic, later examined the claims of Long and admitted that Long had performed the first operation.[152] The question of which man made the discovery is relatively unimportant. What is important is the fact that experimentation had been carried on and that Warren's successful operation gave the profession and the public a valuable medical adjunct.

Once ether was incorporated in materia medica, its exact application had to be determined. J. B. Beck laid down seven rules for its administration: (1) the patient should not take food before ether; (2) the mind should be calm and composed; (3) those present at the operation should be quiet while administering ether; (4) a sponge impregnated with ether should be placed near the mouth and the inhalation should be rapid and deep, but if chloroform were used, breathing should be slower; (5) there should be an ample

[151] *Ibid.*, p. 17; Gross, *19th Century Physicians*, pp. 811-812.

[152] Atkinson, *op. cit.*, pp. 149-159; this is the best exposition of Long's case.

supply of air; (5) one person and one person only should have charge of anesthetics; and (7) the patient should not be shocked upon his return to consciousness. He felt that the use of ether was desirable in midwifery, delirium tremens, puerperal convulsions, spasmodic asthma, idiopathic tetanus and neuralgia.[153]

Besides ether, chloroform became popular as an anesthetic. Independently discovered by Dr. Samuel Guthrie of Sacketts Harbor in 1831 at the same time that experimentation was going forward in European countries, in 1847 its proper use was developed by Dr. Simpson of Edinburgh.[154] The curiosity of the profession regarding anesthesia appeared in an account of an amputation performed in Wabash County, Illinois, and reported in the *American Journal of Medical Sciences* in 1849.

Consultation having been premised, and amputation determined on, the patient was placed upon a table, in a recumbent posture, his head and shoulders reposing on pillows, the Tourniquet, &c., arranged; when we proceeded to exhibit a small teaspoonful of chloroform, in a sponge to his mouth and nostrils; but in a little more than a minute he became sick and vomited, and the sponge was removed during his effort to vomit, and the chloroform having measurably if not entirely escaped, it was again charged with the same quantity and exhibited as before, when vomiting again occurred. The above circumstances were repeated, and inhalation carried on with short intermissions, during which, several drachms of the chloroform were consumed. The time occupied by this exhibition was nine minutes and thirty seconds, when the patient assumed the appearance of sound sleep. [The surgeon then amputated, and when the patient, two minutes later regained consciousness] Dr. Rounolds inquired of him whether he was still desirous of

[153] Beck, J. B., *Lectures on Materia Medica and Therapeutics* (N. Y., 1851), pp. 419-422.
[154] *On the Progress of Recent Science*, p. 18.

having his thigh amputated, and he replied that he was, and hoped that we would not keep him longer in suspense. On being informed that the operation was completed, and that nothing remained but to dress the stump, he indicated some doubt of the truth of the assertion when some one present elevated his shoulders while I raised the stump, to the evident surprise and pleasure of the patient.

In this case it was learned, as it had been very many times since 1846, that the patient recovered in a very short time, thereby adding another reason for the use of ether or chloroform.[155]

The use of anesthesia aroused the opposition of those who thought it unsafe, of the religious and of those who feared its illegitimate use. Dr. Walter Channing of Boston in *A Treatise on Etherization in Childbirth* answered many objections by citing five hundred and eighty cases wherein it had been useful.[156] One correspondent in the *St. Louis Medical and Surgical Journal* said that

So pleasant, and at the same time so powerful are the exhilarating and anodyne effects of chloroform, that the day is probably not distant when it will not only be used by every physician, but be " hung on some rusty nail " by the side of paregoric and Godfrey's cordial in every place and every log cabin in the land, and that for one dose of either of the latter articles a hundred delightful sniffs will be taken from the former. If a little child has a belly ache or an old woman a face ache, a few pleasant whiffs from the green bottle will dissipate it all—and when the pipe or the quid fail to drive away devils or bring angels to minister to the hypochondriac or the hysteric, a few inhalations from a fashionable pocket

[155] *American Journal of Medical Sciences*, N. S. XVII, 1849, pp. 91-92.
[156] *Ibid.*, N. S. XVII, pp. 99-116.

THE PRACTICE OF PHYSICK 145

inhaler will accomplish both—make ugliness beauty, and transport from hell to heaven without a change of heart.[157]

Operations were usually performed in the home of the patient due to the scarcity of hospitals and also to the poor reputations of those which did exist. In amputation there was modification of procedure during the first half of the nineteenth century. The patient was strapped upon the table, the good leg fastened down, the turniquet applied and the operation begun. After a double incision, linen was used to keep the wound open, and, when the bone broke, nippers removed the broken bits. When the operation was completed, blood vessels were ligated, the flesh and muscles piled over the stump and a cap placed over it which remained untouched for three days.[158]

Hygienic precautions did not particularly disturb the doctor or his patient. The idea that disease came from the atmosphere led Mott to recommend spring and autumn as the best seasons and morning as the best time of the day to operate without fear of infection.[159] The attitude of the profession is well illustrated by a quotation from an account of an operation for uterine tumor in which the surgeon found that " the remaining part could be separated from the uterus as a distinct substance; still as it was not supplied with nerves, the great part was torn off by the finger nail." The patient died.[160]

Once the operation was performed, tying arteries and veins became important. Dr. A. H. Stevens of New York suggested various methods for tying these. The broad flat

[157] *Saint Louis Medical and Surgical Journal*, ed. by M. L. Linton (8 volumes, 1843-1850, St. Louis, 1843-1850), VIII, p. 315.

[158] Cooper, Samuel, *The First Lines of the Practice of Surgery...* (Phila., 1808) (4th American Ed. 7th Eng. 1844), pp. 424-429.

[159] Mott, *Velpeau*, I, pp. 9-11.

[160] *Boston Medical and Surgical Journal*, VIII, 1833, p. 69.

ligature gradually gave way to the practice of passing a crooked needle around the artery or vein. Ligatures were usually waxed thread, flaxen thread or silk, since the gut or " animal matter " was apt to result in abscess. Stevens advised tying as near the vascular connexion as possible.[161] Occasionally the wound was scarified by means of oil of turpentine after a cataplasm in order to prevent gangrene. Finally the wound was dressed with dry lint.[162]

After ligatures (or as some doctors recommended before the ligatures), it was necessary to dress the wound. Mott summarizing the best practice stated that he cleansed the wound with small balls of lint or with a sponge soaked in tepid water, then made the ligatures and united the edges by adhesive tape, and then bandaged with soft and narrow bandages, leaving the wound a chance to drain. Other methods which he noted, were the open or German dressing by which wet packs were kept on the wound, a practice which he considered useful in summer but dangerous in other seasons and the dressings which allowed the wound to unite after drainage.[163] The bandages were made of linen, calico, woolen, rubber, thread, riband, roller, wet and glutinous or adhesive.[164] There were many types of bandages: the T, three-tailed, four-tailed, many-tailed, single and double-headed, retention, expulsive and united.[165] Although bandaging the wound was customary later in the period, Dr. Physick, a famous American surgeon of the early nineteenth century, kept the wound open seven or eight days in winter and two or three days in summer by means of removing the dressing every two days to allow it to heal from the

[161] *The Medical and Surgical Register* (3 volumes, 1818-1820, N. Y., 1818-1820), eds. John Watts, V. Mott and A. H. Stevens, I, pp. 61-65.
[162] Sharp, *op. cit.*, p. 28.   [163] Mott, *Velpeau*, I, pp. 52-61.
[164] *Ibid.*, I, pp. 116-127.   [165] Druitt, *op. cit.*, pp. 487-488.

THE PRACTICE OF PHYSICK 147

bottom.[166] Stitches did not require bandaging, but the wound was covered with lint soaked in ointment.[167]

In hemorrhages the tourniquet was applied wherever possible, or the arteries were ligated. Compressing the sides of the wound so that small vessels could be brought together to stop the bleeding was also common. Algaric, which is similar to sponge, was used to fill up the wound and close surrounding vessels when hemorrhage began. Although in small hemorrhages styptic, cold air, water wine spirits, alum and blue vitriol were used, actual cautery, excepting in the mouth, and caustic, even though popular, were banned by the medical authorities.[168]

However much the profession was theoretically prepared to operate, it is doubtful that surgery played the part in this period that it does today. Lacking anesthesia and aseptic surgery, doctors were reluctant to resort to operations. Such operations as were performed, as the discussion of instruments demonstrates, were limited to amputations, to the removal of stones from the abdomen, of foreign matter from the eye, and of tumors and abscesses, and to such minor efforts as bandaging wounds. Occasionally daring attempts were made, such as the operations of Mott, McDowell and Simms, but the average practitioner rarely turned from medication to surgery. Students in the medical schools were given little training in surgery. The student, Boardman, complained that there was not one operative case in the Geneva College infirmary.[169] Although the number of surgeons did increase during these years, none of them could become a real specialist until the profession understood the significance of anesthesia and aseptic surgery.

[166] Gibson, W., *The Institutions and Practice of Surgery*... (2 volumes, Phila., 1827) (7th Ed., Phila., 1845), II, pp. 410-411.

[167] Ferguson, Sir W., *A System of Practical Surgery*. Notes and additional illustrations by G. W. Norris (Phila., 1845), p. 52.

[168] Cooper, S., *op. cit.*, pp. 42-54.   [169] *Cf. supra*, p. 90.

CHAPTER V

MEDICAL ETHICS AND FEES

WE may now turn our attention to the doctor's relations with his fellows. Gradually, the medical men of colonial times had approached a professional attitude. As their numbers grew and their medical contacts increased through the formation of societies and the circulation of magazines, they felt the need of rules to govern their activities as members of a profession.

Oddly enough, Percival's work, the best and most complete code of ethics, was in existence before 1800. Whether or not the old practitioners knew of this work, they felt its influence upon the professionally-minded of their group and in the by-laws of the medical societies. Occasionally these by-laws developed into codes of ethics, such as the *Boston Medical Police* of 1808, which, relying almost entirely upon Percival, enjoyed popularity throughout New England. The textbooks and teachers in the courses in medical jurisprudence emphasized the requirements of professional etiquette, and it was here that the professors had their chance to build *esprit de corps*. The work which, eventually, became authoritative was the *American Medical Association Code of Medical Ethics*, published after the formation of that body in 1846. Dr. Isaac Hays, speaking for the committee which framed the work, stated that they had followed Percival's earlier work to the extent, at times, of using his actual words, and had relied upon Rush for most of the other material.[1]

[1] *American Medical Association, Code of Ethics of . . . Adopted May, 1847.*

Medical behavior in America, during the greater part of the period from the Revolution to 1850, was dominated by the English physician, Thomas Percival, through his book, *Medical Jurisprudence or Code of Ethics and Institutes adopted by the Profession of Physic and Surgery.* Other books on medical jurisprudence came out, among them T. R. Beck's, but so far as ethics was concerned Percival was commonly accepted. The by-laws of the societies were few, and merely simplified or elaborated statements by Percival. Occasionally, *Police* or codes of ethics were issued by societies, such as the New Hampshire Medical Society's *Police.* Undoubtedly, the opinions of professors in the colleges often did much to shape the minds of young medical students. Rush, whose speeches, as we have seen, contained much sound advice, and other eminent physicians could not have failed to send out young doctors with a professional attitude.

Percival's book, which was published in America in 1794, treated: *The Professional conduct relating to Hospitals, or other Medical Charities; Of Professional conduct in Private and General Practice; Of the Conduct of Physicians toward Apothecaries; and, Of the Knowledge of Law requisite for Physicians and Surgeons.* With regard to the conduct of doctors in hospitals and charities, thirty rules were stated. The physician's and surgeon's first duty was to maintain his position without offending the patient. The poor as well as rich should receive the chance of consultation in hospitals; but in dispensaries, because of the touchiness and lack of breeding of paupers, a combination of kindliness and authoritative manner was advised. The profession should respect the patient's feelings and emotions by not discussing his case in his presence or asking questions in such a tone as to be overheard by other patients. The solemn duties of reminding patients of their wills and having a clergyman present to remind them of the next world fell upon the doctor. The staff was admonished to use only drugs of the best quality. Members of the staff were to refrain from telling derogatory anecdotes about their fellows. All charges were centered in the staff and subject to the staff's opinion. Because of the separation into the surgical and general-physician departments a careful check on which group was to handle cases had to be maintained. Percival emphasized care in trying new remedies, accuracy in accounts of all cases, effective and rapid cure and judicious segregation of cases to prevent contagion.

The hospital staff was to meet at least once a month to discuss the affairs of the institution. In consultation the junior officers gave their opinions first, but the doctor in charge of the case was not required to follow the decision of the majority. In all cases where surgeons and physicians conferred, surgeons gave their opinions first, which might imply that in Percival's mind surgeons were inferior, a fact certainly not true in America. Due notice of consultation was required, and outsiders were admitted only by unanimous vote. He declared against "operative days", that is days set aside for operations, and added that twenty-four hours' notice of operations should be given. Spectators should be admitted only with the consent of the patient, and on condition of absolute silence. Likewise, he stressed cleanly dress and instruments in all surgical cases. Venereal disease in women required exceptional privacy. Then followed a number of rules regarding the insane, pointing out the need of tenderness (this was in 1794) in all cases excepting mania, in which firmness was ordered, and finally requesting more careful collection of data in mental disease.[2]

[2] Percival, Thomas, *Medical Jurisprudence or a Code of Ethics* ... (1794), pp. 3-23.

With regard to the doctor's conduct in general practice, Percival gave the consensus of professional opinion. Secrecy, care and "reasonable indulgence" with regard to each other were the major rules. Doctors had to be strictly temperate in drinking. Pessimism on the part of doctors was bad. "Officious interference in a case under the charge of another should be avoided." If a doctor was called on a case, it was his duty to consult the doctor previously in charge. "In large and opulent towns, the *distinction* between the provinces of *physic* and *surgery* should be steadily maintained." While consultations were always helpful, special consultation was to be limited and the fee doubled. In these consultations the order of opinion was the same as in hospitals. Although education was the best means of preparing a man for the practice of physic, a self-made doctor was not to be excluded. Doctors were told to be punctual at consultations and to avoid giving new prognostications. To keep the respect of the poor, doctors were advised to limit the number of visits, but for the moral effect, to continue them in hopeless cases. If a doctor took over the practice of another for a long period, he could collect the fees; but if the time was short, he was not to collect. Each town should have its medical rates, although doctors usually should give free attention to clergy and each other.[3] Doctors were to demand double pay for letters of advice. It is the duty, he wrote, of each doctor to discourage the use of quack medicines. All regular practitioners had to give discoveries to the profession instead of developing them as secret nostrums. To maintain professional dignity, quarrels should be settled by the profession instead of allowing them to become public property through newspapers.[4]

[3] *Cf. infra*, Chapter VII, p. 225, with regard to the clergy.
[4] Percival, *op. cit.*, pp. 23-36.

In Percival's advice regarding the conduct of a physician towards apothecaries an old antagonism appears. Although the doctor was told to familiarize the apothecary with the case, he was advised to condescend to the latter and personally to examine all drugs. The ignorance, especially of the country apothecary, required guidance and kindliness from the regular profession. Somewhat inconsistently, he concluded with a word of pity for apothecaries, because their profits were so small.[5]

It is interesting, by contrast, to examine the *Code of Ethics of the Philadelphia College of Pharmacy*, which appeared in the American Medical Association report for 1848. Apothecaries were to refrain from prescribing and from furthering the interests of any one doctor. Although they might sell patent medicines, they were not to manufacture them. A set rate of charges was to be maintained in each community. Errors of doctors as well as those of fellow druggists, unless caused by ignorance, were to be kept from patients. Sales of impure drugs were to be punished, and the sale of poisons to be closely controlled. Finally a four-year apprenticeship and two years of formal study were proposed to raise the standard of apothecaries.[6] The spirit of cooperation reflects a much different attitude from that of Percival in his advice to doctors on their relation to apothecaries. It is explainable by the fact that by 1848 the two were no longer invading each other's field to augment their meager incomes.

The need of making a living brought up other problems. The New York Medical Society in its code of 1823 forbade certain practices of indigent members:

[5] *Ibid.*, pp. 36-43.
[6] A. M. A. *Transactions*, 1848, pp. 297-301.

A physician in indigent circumstances is not permitted to embrace or exercise any business which would degrade the character of his profession, such as keeping a tavern, lottery office, gambling, victualling, or play-house. Any low trade or servile, mercenary occupation is incompatible with the dignity and independence of medical avocation. In such extreme and derogatory situations a physician forfeits the privileges of his profession.[7]

Since the desire of members of the profession for larger incomes led to such practices, the Philadelphia Medical Society in 1843 forbade any member to publish his qualifications, to deal in patent medicines, to report any part of his practice in lay publications and to practise or sanction "any system of quackery or imposture, including what is called homœopathia."[8]

Despite the efforts of professionally-minded physicians, there is much evidence that Percival and other authors of codes depicted ideal rather than actual conditions. Speaking in 1818 at Dartmouth, Professor N. D. Mussey said:

The remark has often been made, that physicians are seldom heard to speak well of each other. This remark is usually accompanied with the query, Why is it that a spirit of jealousy and hostility is so widely diffused among the faculty of medicine?[9]

As late as 1849, Rush Van Dyke stated:

Nothing, perhaps, has injured the profession more, in the public estimation, than the petty envy, jealousy, and uncharitableness which formerly characterized the manners and feelings

---

[7] *New York Medical Society, 1807-1831*, pp. 232-233.
[8] *Boston Medical and Surgical Journal*, XXVIII, 1843, p. 303.
[9] Mussey, N. D., *Address Read to the Medical Class at Dartmouth, 1818*, p. 16 (Pamphlet Collection, Library of the University of Pennsylvania).

of its members. A few years ago, very few physicians, either in towns or country places, were on friendly terms and so far was this feeling of animosity carried, that professors in the same schools, of the highest rank in their respective branches, have refused, the one to enter the ward of an hospital while the other was present, or to hold any communication with each other except such as their official position as teachers peremptorily demanded, in faculty meeting.[10]

After reading such remarks by members of the profession, we may conclude that medical ethics were not observed so carefully one hundred years ago as they are today. Various reasons account for this condition. The college term was not long enough to inculcate a professional attitude. During most of the period there was no state or national body powerful enough to protect professional ethics. Expulsion from existing organizations seldom meant disgrace, and the public accorded many quacks a hearty welcome. Finally, observance of any rules was a luxury which few individuals, crowded by competitors, could afford. Although the general practitioner could not always live up to the codes, there were many doctors with large income and high standards who did. Among such men were Benjamin Rush, Philip S. Physick, Wright Post, Valentine Mott, Nathan Smith Davis, David Hosack and Richard Arnold, to name only a few, whose conduct both toward the general public and their fellow practitioners will favorably compare with that of present-day physicians.

MEDICAL FEES

While the medical profession was accepting Percival as the dictator in matters of behavior, it was also developing, locally, a set rate of charges for its services. Undoubtedly

---

[10] Van Dyke, Rush, *Valedictory Address to Graduates of Philadelphia College of Medicine, 1849* (Phila., 1849), pp. 9-10.

the profession had fixed such rates in colonial times, but charges endorsed by members of a society or locality did not become common until after the Revolution. Besides the fact that there were few societies in which such tables of fees could be arranged and maintained, there was popular distrust of medical men and what might be interpreted as their efforts for monopolistic rates. Virginia, as early as 1736, objected to fixed rates and determined all charges by a law, the preamble of which stated: " WHEREAS the practice of phisic in this colony, is most commonly taken up and followed, by surgeons, apothecaries, or such as have only served apprenticeships to those trades, who often prove very unskilful in the art of a phisician; and yet do demand excessive fees."[11] Bowing before such feeling the medical societies of New York, New Hampshire and the District of Columbia forbade tables of rates,[12] although many counties and towns in New York State had them.

In the study of these charges it is necessary to remember that the doctor listed only *minimum* charges. The necessity of taking care of the poor and accepting a meager return, if any, was a burden upon the profession required by humanitarian considerations. When the members could find some rich patients as compensation, the care of the poor was less burdensome. Before examining charges throughout the country, it is best to recall that not all doctors approved the set charge, among them Rush, who in 1789 said,

[11] *Virginia, The Statutes at Large...of...1619-1792;* Comp. of William Walter Hening (13 volumes, various places, 1810-1823), IV, 1736, pp. 509-510.

[12] *Med. Soc. State of New York, 1807-1831,* 1808, p. 13; *The Charter, By-Laws, Regulations and Police of the New-Hampshire Medical Society* (Concord, 1822), p. 20; *History of the Medical Society of the District of Columbia, 1817-1909* (Washington, 1909), the last stated that the Medical Association of the District was organized in 1833 to make a fee-table possible, p. 14.

"On the contrary, let the number and *time* of your visits, the nature of your patient's disease, and his rank in his family or society, determine the figures in your account." [13]

The first fee bill of which there is record was adopted by the Medical Society of New Jersey in 1766.[14] Although the *Boston Medical Police* of 1864 states that the first fee bill was established there in 1788, the account book of John Warren of that city contains a list of charges in his handwriting, entitled the "List of fees of the Boston Medical Society" and dated May 1782.[15] The doctors of New York City made such a list in 1790 which was translated into terms of American currency in 1798 and reaffirmed in 1816.[16] After 1800 many tables appeared in the charters and by-laws of medical societies, although there were continued complaints of the regular practitioners against cheap doctors and the lack of tables of charges.[17]

It is interesting to study charges in the various cities and sections of the country. According to the Boston *Fee-Bill* of 1788, the charge for a visit was four shillings, or sixty-seven cents. Ten years later this fee and others had risen about fifty percent, with the visit charge at one dollar. In 1808 the rising cost of living as well as the mounting wealth of the town led to a visit charge of $1.50, and other increases, reductions being permitted for persons in mod-

---

[13] Rush, *op. cit.*, I, p. 399.

[14] New Jersey Medical Society, *op. cit.*, pp. 9-13.

[15] *Boston Medical Police for 1864* (Boston, 1864), pp. 14-16; John C. Warren Day Book, 1781-1791. Mss. in Boston Medical Library; other Day Books are in the Massachusetts Historical Society Library. This is the elder Warren.

[16] The table of charges for 1790 is in the New York Historical Society Library.

[17] *Boston Medical Intelligencer*, II, p. 151, gives a good example of the complaints.

erate circumstances. Thereafter there was little change.[18] Other charges listed by Warren in 1782 were for midwifery, two pounds eight shillings, for venereal cases six pounds, for capital operations five pounds, for rising in the night one pound four shillings, for decoctions three shillings, for pills and powders eight shillings per dozen, and for electuaries three shillings.[19] In 1817 the Boston Medical Association regulated as follows: members were forbidden contact with irregulars; they were forbidden to make family contracts (that is, agreements to care for a family by the year); they were to report all irregularities.[20] The Fee-Bill, drawn at the same time, opened with the following statement:

The following table contains the lowest fees, which shall be charged for the services, to which they are respectively annexed; but in proportion to the importance of the case and the advice offered, or in consequence of an extraordinary attendance, the charge shall be increased; and the members of this Association consider themselves bound to increase their charges agreeably to this rule.[21]

These charges, which had the endorsement of at least the leading physicians of the city, were $2 to $5 for the first visit and $1.50 for subsequent visits. A consultation visit was $5 and subsequent consultation, $3. Differentiation was made, as was common in all such tables, between night and day visits, with night visits at $5 or night advice at the doctor's home, $3. Again, rates varied according to distance and neighborhood. Other charges were: midwif-

[18] *Boston Medical Police for 1864*, pp. 14-16.
[19] Warren, Day Book, 1781-1791.
[20] *Boston Medical Association, Rules and Regulations of* ... (Boston, 1817), p. 5.
[21] *Ibid.*, p. 6.

ery during the day, $12, at night, $15; capital operations, such as amputations of large limbs, lithotomy, trepanning and extirpation of large tumors, $40; specific rates for operations included fistua in ano, $20; tapping for dropsy and reducing luxations or fractures of large bones, $10; amputation of fingers or toes, and excision of small tumors, $8; reducing luxations or fractures of small bones, stitching wounds, opening large abscesses and similar operations, $5; passing a catheter, $5; venesection in addition to a visit, $1; extraction of a tooth, $1, when at the surgeon's home, and $1.50 at the patient's home. Vaccination was $5. Gonorrhea was treated for $10 and "all other cases of syphilis" were $15. No mention was made of powders, pills and such prescriptions.[22]

The New York City *Fee-Bill* of 1816, a renewal of that of 1790, was similar to Boston's, differing in the greater latitude of charges and the inclusion of more items. With regard to visits the charges and various allowances were made for distance from the physician's home. This table included verbal advice at $5 and a letter of advice from $10 to $15. Bleeding charges were: by cupping glasses, $5; at the arm, $2; and at the jugular vein, $5. Dressing a blister was $1; scarifying the eye was $5. Rates for fractures allowed the doctor more discretion, reduction of a simple fracture being between $10 and $20, compound fractures being $30. Dislocations, depending upon their nature, were from $5 to $20, setting the hip-joint being from $30 to $50. Operations for reduction of hernia cost from $10 to $25. Amputations depended upon the member and were: breast, $50; leg, $50; at hip or shoulder joint, $100 to $150; finger or toe, $10 (as against $8 charged in Boston). Extractions which included other items than teeth, were

[22] *Ibid.*, pp. 6-7.

graded as follows: eye, $100; testes, $50; tonsils, $25; a polypus, $25; and a tumor, from $5 to $50. The fee for perforating the rectum was $25, while the fees for perforating the nostrils, external ear, vagina or urethra were from $5 to $25. Paracentesis of the abdomen cost from $5 to $25, and in the thorax, $50. Operations for tic douloureux and harelip were $25; hernia, $125; anal fistula, $50; wry neck, $50. Operations for cataract by depression was $125 and by extraction, $150. The cost of removal of aneurisms depended upon location, those upon the external iliac artery being $200 and those upon the posterior tibial only $25. Specific charges were: lithotomy, $150; circumcision, $10. A tooth extraction at the patient's home was $2 and at the surgeon's home, $1. Midwifery was much more expensive in New York than in Boston, its charges being from $25 to $35 in common cases and $35 to $60 in tedious or difficult cases. The penalties for social diseases were greater, gonorrhea being from $15 to $30 and syphilis from $25 to $100.[28]

Boston and New York represent the highest charges made in the country. Philadelphia, although a city with medical talent unsurpassed in America, or perhaps because of the competition of so much talent, did not have high rates. Writing in 1842, a correspondent of the *Boston Medical and Surgical Journal* said:

[28] New York City Medical Association, May, Part II, pp. 126-127, 1816; the reason for giving this list of rates rather than those of 1790 is that the charges in 1790 were stated in terms of English money. This New York table also included pharmaceutical charges. Some were: single prescription, $.50; pills, per dozen, $.75; bolus, each, $.50; electuaries, per ounce, $1; infusions, per pound, $2; tinctures, per ounce, $.50. ointments and cerates, per ounce, $.50; blistering plasters, according to size, $.50 to $2.50; decoctions, per pound, $2; single medicine dispensed without a visit, $1; an anodyne draught, $.50; and preparation and administration of an enema, $2.

There [Philadelphia] fees are very moderate, and complained of by themselves. I was told repeatedly that scarcely any man, however distinguished, charges over one dollar a visit in ordinary practice. This is the regular charge in such places as Albany, Troy, Utica, and New Haven. In New York and Boston, men of similar distinction charge decidedly higher; one dollar and a half in Boston and two dollars in New York being the common charge of fashionable practitioners.[24]

The fee bill of the College of Physicians of Philadelphia, an organization whose members were the outstanding physicians of the city, in 1834, bears out this statement. Vaccination was $5 and re-vaccination from $2 to $3; reducing fractures and luxations were $5 to $10; passing the catheter was from $1 to $5; anal fistula was $20 to $40. All of these rates are lower or have lower limits than the charges in the other two cities. The charge for midwifery, however, was from $8 to $20, which was as high as the rate in Boston, but lower than that in New York.[25]

The position of Washington as the national capital makes its code of interest. Furthermore, Congress, more than the various state legislatures, protected the medical profession. The Medical Association, in 1833, set the following rates: visit and prescription, $1; consultation visit, $5; or if beyond the city limits, $8, with subsequent visits, $2. Venesection, the extraction of a tooth, prescriptions, dressing a wound, all cost $1. Passing a catheter during a visit was $5, but if it was often repeated, only $2. Visits for every mile beyond the center of the city were $2 additional to the ordinary fee. Night attendance was from $5 to $10. Specific attendance or cures for gonorrhea were $10; syphilis, $15; midwifery, in the day $12, and in the night, $15; capital

[24] *Boston Medical and Surgical Journal*, XXVI, 1842, p. 28.
[25] *College of Physicians of Philadelphia, Charter, Ordinance, and By-Laws of the* ... (Phila., 1834), p. 17.

operations were from $40 to $100; fractures or luxations, fistula and tapping for dropsy were $10; minor amputations were $5; stitching recent wounds, opening abscesses, introducing a seton or issue were $3, with $2 for subsequent dressings; vaccination was $3.[26] This fee bill was accompanied by a statement to the effect that rates might be reduced for the poor, any payment being acceptable, and might be raised according to the difficulties attending treatment.[27]

In small towns, the fees were much lower. Lowell, Massachusetts, is an example. Visits were charged at $.75 for the first mile and $.40 for each subsequent mile. Night visits brought $.25 per mile in addition. Office advice cost $.25, office treatment, $.50; venesection, $.75 on a visit and $.50 at the office. An office dressing was $.50, with subsequent dressings $.25 each. A tooth extraction was $.50. Consultation visits were $1.50, and $1 for subsequent visits. Midwifery was $5 per case. Rates were higher for major operations: amputations, $30; trepanning, $38; lithotomy, $50; but fistula only $5. Fractures were: for thigh $10 and for all others, $5. Removal of a testicle was $25; harelip, $10; fingers or toes, $1. Abscesses were removed for $.50; small tumors, $1. Vaccination was $.50. Gonorrhea treatment was $5 while syphilis treatment was $10.[28]

Other fee bills from rural communities, such as those of Washington County, New York and Belmont County, Ohio, as well as the rates of Kentucky physicians, show slight variations from the Lowell schedules.[29] Samuel D. Gross

[26] *Regulation and System of Ethics of the Medical Association of Washington* (Washington, 1837), p. 5.

[27] *Ibid.*, p. 6.

[28] *Lowell Medical Association, Charter, By-Laws and Regulations of* ... (1837), p. 37.

[29] *Boston Medical and Surgical Journal*, XVIII, 1838, pp. 50-51; Belmont Medical Society (Ohio), *Proceedings*, 1847, pp. 12-14; *Journal*

in his *Autobiography* gives similar fees which he charged at Easton, Pennsylvania, early in the century: town visits, $.50; out of town, $1 to $2; consultation, $5 for the first time and $1 subsequently; obstetrics, $5 for the poor and $10 to $25 for the wealthy. In Cincinnati, which was a larger town, the fee for a visit was $1 and for a consultation, $5.[30] The rates in use in New Jersey, while not so high as those in Washington, were higher than the fees which Gross charged.

In Niagara County, New York, the medical society drew up rates for the poor. Visits, including ordinary medicine, were $.625; every mile over one-half mile were $.125; night mileage was $.75 per mile; setting a thigh bone was $3; midwifery, $3. This table, the only evidence of set charges for the poor, was not accepted by other doctors of the state.[31]

Turning our attention to other sections of the country, we find fewer fee bills. South Carolina, in 1850, adopted again the bill which had been drawn up in 1792, which in turn seems to have been a revision of one for 1755. The terms of the English monetary system were given American values but do not seem to have been raised. This list was the most complete, covering all fields of medical attention. In some cases, such as for visits, the rates were about one-half the level in New York and Boston. The range of charges, however, was wide, such as $4.67 to $13.98 for advice by letter. Consultations were $13.98. For powders, pills and similar medicines the charges were around $.20. Major operations did not exceed $50, a minimum rather

of the *Proceedings of a Committee of Physicians of Kentucky* (1841), pp. 17-18.

[30] Gross, *Autobiography*, pp. 152-153.

[31] New York Medical Society, *Proceedings, 1841-1843* (Albany, 1843), App., pp. 62-63.

than a maximum limit in New York and Boston. Oddly enough, inoculation was $13.98 and vaccination $5 to $9, which probably was caused by the difficulty in preserving variolous matter or vaccine. Midwifery also was more expensive, common cases being between $30 and $50, prolonged cases, $50 to $80. The use of instruments increased the charge to $80 or $100. Advice to the midwife was $30. This table was also organized better than any other table in use. Classifications were natural and complete and their length gave doctors little chance to plead ignorance of professional charges.[32]

By 1843, charges in the Southwest had reached tabular form. Prescriptions, venesection and extracting teeth were $1; cupping and leeching, $2; preparing and administering a dose of medicine, $.50; travel per mile during the day was $1; at night, $2; a town visit or call while in the country was $1; detention over an hour, each $1, night detention being $2 per hour; consultation fees were from $10 to $20 (explainable no doubt by the distance traveled). Obstetrical cases were from $10 to $25; important surgical operations were $50 and minor operations from $5 to $20; setting bones, depending upon the fracture and its location, were from $15 to $25; and dressing wounds, from $2 to $5.[33]

At an earlier date, 1825, the *New England Journal of Medicine and Surgery* published the following discussion of the table in use in Mississippi and Lousiana:

[32] *South Carolina, Constitution and By-Laws of the Medical Society of* ... (Charleston, 1850), pp. 65-69. A Recipe Book, 1812-1813, author unknown, in the Boston Medical Library contains this fee table of 1792 and the supplement of 1804. The tables are not so complete but the charges are substantially the same.

[33] *Boston Medical and Surgical Journal*, XXVIII, 1843, p. 319.

A fee table contains one regulation which is a very important one, and goes to make up the benefits they secure to the profession and public. They require a regular settlement of accounts between the parties, and generally prescribe that accounts should be rendered, and, if possible, closed, once a year. The good effects of this is universally felt and acknowledged. A man who received the reward of his services learns something of their value. If he be a prudent man, he will arrive at competence and a profession which will do this for him, will be cultivated by himself, and be respected by others. The competence is the fruit of great sacrifices and great benefits, and will neither be envied or contemned. In this part of the country, with the exception of a very few places, it is in no degree the custom to settle professional accounts at any particular period. The common practice is to let them alone, and suffer them to accumulate indefinitely. When something is wanted by the physician which money might procure, the farmer or trader, a debtor patient, is asked to supply the occasion *in kind*. This is always done where it is convenient. The article and its value are charged. This goes on, and the case has occurred in which upon the settlement of a physician's books, in consequence of death or otherwise, he is debtor instead of creditor, with a considerable amount due him on his own books. Now this is not well. It is well neither for the profession or the public. It makes the support of the physician very much a matter of accident, and it diminishes the wider influence which he, as a man of learning and of reputation, should exert about him.[34]

This statement probably expressed the attitude of the whole profession on this system of payment. Much as the profession desired to standardize its charges and regularize collections, there were always physicians who preferred to let matters take their own course or who, because of the very economy of frontier farming and plantation life, had no other choice.

[34] *New England Journal of Medicine and Surgery*, XIV, 1825, pp. 53-54.

These fee tables represent the charges throughout the country,[35] but they give no indication of the difficulty of collecting cash for services. An examination of account books, especially of those in the Boston Medical Library, reveals the universality of payments in kind. From them one learns the exchange values of goods. For instance, William Sweat (Hollis, New Hampshire) cancelled fourteen debts to the extent of $60.85 by accepting hay in payment at the rate of $2.50 for a "half ton clover hay", $3.00 for a "half ton of good hay" and $5.00 for a ton of hay. Samuel Hayes (New Jersey) accepted a barrel of flour and granted $5.75 credit. Dr. Daniel Pierce (possibly of Boston) allowed a patient, Robert Breir, to work off his account at an average wage of three shillings a day, between 1791 and 1800. Barter was not limited to unknown doctors. It enabled physicians of prominence, who enjoyed large incomes, to collect outstanding accounts. In a note dated May 24, 1851, Dr. Jacob Bigelow referred to an arrangement with one Eben Sears whereby he furnished Mr. Sears and his family with medical attention and the latter did odd-jobs for him. They passed receipts, and upon the death of Mr. Sears the debts nearly cancelled each other. Other account books indicate that such an arrangement was not exceptional. They also show agreement with the fee tables of their districts.[36]

Besides barter, family contracts were frowned upon by the profession. This system was the subject of an attack in the New York Medical Society as late as 1850. Exact evidence of its existence is missing, since the doctor's books were often carelessly kept and the bill sent at the end of the

[35] For a complete list of the fee-tables which I have used, see Bibliography, p. 257.

[36] For a list of the Account Books, Day Books and other records which I have used, see Bibliography, pp. 255-256.

year might merely represent a general idea by the doctor of his services. This may explain the note of Joseph Parrish to the effect that he had received fifty dollars " in full for Medical and Surgical attendance " on the family of Whittier Evens, in 1811.[37] Doctors refer to family contracts as a common practice, and one can easily understand its development on the plantations of the South; but such conclusions are by inference rather than actual proof. The general custom of accepting what a man could afford to pay on his bill naturally interfered with full collection and explains many of the " round numbers " which appear in the account books.

The overcrowded profession resulted in small incomes among the majority of physicians. The *Boston Medical and Surgical Journal,* interesting itself in the size and income of the profession, found that in 1831 New York State had 2549 physicians as against 1742 practicing attorneys and 1300 clergymen.[38] In Chicago in 1838 there were forty physicians for 8000 people; Cincinnati, in 1839, had 100 physicians for a population of 50,000, or one physician for every 500 persons.[39] It is no wonder that an article in this magazine in reply to an exaggeration of the average city practice should say:

But this gentleman is not alone in over-estimating the medical business of a city. The fact is, there are dozens of doctors in all great towns, who scarcely see a patient from Christmas-time to Christmas-time. There are prodigious Ramadams in the receipts of every physician engaged in city practice. As a general rule, there is not a broken bone a-piece, in a twelve-month, notwithstanding the exalted ideas of our

[37] Etting Collection, Physicians, p. 75.
[38] *Boston Medical and Surgical Journal,* IV, 1831, p. 184.
[39] *Ibid.,* XVI, 1838, p. 387; XX, 1839, p. 395.

southern friend, in relation to the amount and universal profit arising from the art chirurgical. If it requires a long and thorough drilling to succeed at all in the country, a man is compelled to labor patiently, many years, in a city, before he can command his daily bread in exchange for prescriptions.[40]

Earlier in 1832, this magazine pointed out that the profession lacked riches because its members did not have the time or opportunity to speculate and because its social purpose kept its members from thoughts of money.[41] The opinion of the Boston weekly was endorsed by its western counter part, *The Western Journal of the Medical and Physical Sciences*, which asked where one might go and not find twice as many lawyers or doctors as were needed, and suggested that most physicians turn to wheat raising.[42] In a commencement address at Yale Medical School, Luther Ticknor held out to the " benevolent enterprising physician " the possibilities of self-support, but little more.[43]

The professors in the medical schools had no cause for complaint, when enrollments reached three and four hundred and each student paid the professor a fee of about fifteen dollars. As a result the incomes of popular professors reached and even occasionally exceeded $8000 yearly, representing great purchasing power.[44] On the other hand, the rural practitioner could not have received more than the $500 yearly income which the *Boston Medical and Surgical Journal* considered normal for the established physician.[45]

[40] *Ibid.*, XV, 1836, p. 273.
[41] *Ibid.*, IV, 1832, pp. 9-10.
[42] *The Western Journal of the Medical and Physical Science* (12 volumes, Cincinnati, 1828-1838), II, p. 495.
[43] Ticknor, Luther, *Annual Address* (Commencement, 1841), p.7.
[44] Cordell, *University of Maryland*, p. 62, states that Granville Pattison received $10,000 a year while there.
[45] *Boston Medical and Surgical Journal*, IX, 1833, p. 112.

Likewise, physicians in charge of state penitentiaries or county jails usually received $500.⁴⁶ This income was sufficient to care for the doctor and his family at that time, for a Hartford practitioner about 1820 managed to save one-half of his $1000 income.⁴⁷

Samuel D. Gross, who was one of the more successful physicians of the period, recorded in his *Autobiography* that his income from his first year's practice was $1400 and that, in addition, he made $500 at the Medical College of Ohio.⁴⁸ He had a personal fortune of $60,000 in 1856, then a sum sufficient to allow luxurious living.⁴⁹ R. D. Arnold, of Savannah, who was successful politically as well as professionally, has left us statements which throw light upon his income. Writing to his wife in 1839, he said:

It runs me almost crazy to think that with hundreds upon hundreds due me professionally I find the greatest difficulty in raising a simple fifty dollars. I hope as I grow old I will grow wiser in money matters & not, with an annual income of over three thousand dollars, be constantly in want of a twenty dollar bill.⁵⁰

Evidently he did reform, for in 1846 he wrote a Savannah planter, Mr. Jacob Waldburg, saying that he had booked $2500 in September alone and added that he intended to make hay while the sun shone.⁵¹

⁴⁶ *Georgia, Acts of ... 1810-1819* (Milledgeville, 1810-1819), 1819, p. 676; *Louisiana, Acts of ...* (New-Orleans, 1820), p. 88 which set the salary for the jail physician in the New Orleans at $400; *Ohio, Statutes of ... in Force, December 7, 1840.* Collated by J. R. Swan (Columbus, 1841), p. 631; *Rhode Island, Public Laws,* rev. ed. 1844 (Providence, 1844), p. 1082.

⁴⁷ Sumner, *Hartford,* p. 22.

⁴⁸ Gross, *Autobiography,* p. 153.

⁴⁹ *Ibid.,* p. 154.

⁵⁰ Arnold, *Letters,* p. 21.

⁵¹ *Ibid.,* p. 30. He became mayor and surrendered the city during the Civil War.

MEDICAL ETHICS AND FEES

Other incomes worth mentioning are those of Amariah Brigham (afterwards superintendent of Utica Asylum for the Insane in New York), who was earning $2500 a year at Hartford in the 1830's.[52] According to George Shattuck's Account Book, this Boston doctor in the lean years following the Panic of 1837, had an income of $9666 in 1838, $8294.50 in 1839 and $9797.50 in 1842.[53] Robert Frary's Day Book showed that his annual receipts between 1822 and 1838 were slightly in excess of $2000.[54] Finally, the Day Book of William Sweat revealed an income of $1019.50 for the year from November 1825 to November 1826.[55] Unfortunately the day books, account books and similar material are those of prominent and successful doctors, and not those of the small country doctor or impoverished city doctor who could hardly afford to keep accounts.

THE SOCIAL POSITION OF THE PROFESSION

We may summarize the status of the American medical profession at this time by saying that, although some members stood well in the esteem of their fellowmen, the great majority did not occupy positions which would favorably compare with those of physicians today.

Any analysis of the factors constituting social position must include birth, wealth, education and the honors bestowed for professional and civic achievements. With regard to birth, the roll of practitioners during this period contains names which are historically significant. In New England alone, there were such names as Warren, Channing, Bigelow, Shattuck, Holyoke and Holmes; in New York, Bard, Mitchill, Hosack and Francis; in Philadelphia, Rush,

---

[52] Gross, *19th Century Physicians*, E. K. Hunt on Brigham, p. 529.
[53] Shattuck's Account Book, 1838-1839 and 1842.
[54] Robert Frary, Day Book, 1822-1838.
[55] Sweat, William, Day-Book, 1825-1831.

Morgan, McClellan, Shippen, Mitchell and Physick; in the South, medicine was a gentleman's profession. On this score the profession would not suffer from comparison with other groups.

While examining medical education, we have seen that a cultural background reflected the student's private interest. In an age when educational institutions were little better than high-class academies, the preparation of the physician compared less favorably with other professional groups than it does today. Few physicians at that time had any collegiate training beyond that necessary for the medical degree.

The third, and probably the most important, factor in determining social position is wealth. It enables a person to sustain a scale of living commensurate with his social propensities. In the study of incomes, we have found many American physicians with yearly incomes sufficient to merit the respect of their fellow men—and automatically to carry with them social prestige. On the other hand the rural doctor often had to supplement his professional income by farming and therefore could not have enjoyed a social position equal to that of the more successful city practitioners.

As a further basis for judgment we have honors accorded physicians. It is significant that these honors, except recognition from the American Philosophical Society, were for work outside the profession. It is true that one hundred years ago people esteemed science; but their esteem was not nearly so great as it is today. During those years, the medical profession developed a scientific attitude. The public, however, eulogizes accomplishment rather than attitude. Although subsequent medical improvements grew out of the new attitude, American physicians, until the 1840's, made no outstanding contributions to human welfare. It follows, therefore, that physicians were honored chiefly for extra-professional activities. When Benjamin Rush died, Thomas Jefferson wrote to John Adams, "'Another of our friends of '76 is gone, another of the co-signers of our country's Independence; and a better man than Rush could not have left us, more benevolent, more learned, of finer genius, or more honest.'"[56] But there is no word regarding his contributions to medical science.

In commenting on the honors accorded American physicians, P. M. Ashburn gives a notable list of public officials and civic leaders, including Samuel Holten, President of Congress in 1780; Arthur Lee, who gave up practice in 1767, and became one of the commissioners to France in 1776; and John Bartlett, who cast the first vote for the Declaration of Independence, was the second signer of that document, and later became Chief Justice and Governor of New Hampshire. Five of the fifty-six signers of the Declaration were doctors, as were twenty-three members of the Provincial Congress of Massachusetts in 1774 and 1775.[57] Samuel L. Mitchill figured prominently in Congress from New York State and in the public affairs of New York City. Samuel Bard was on friendly terms with Washington.[58] John W. Francis was honored by appointments to many societies.[59] When Peter Gansevoort gave a dinner in honor of President Van Buren in 1839, he included Dr. T. R. Beck, author of the book on medical jurisprudence, and James M'Naughton, oftimes president of the state medical society.[60]

[56] Gross, *19th Century Physicians*, p. 46.
[57] Ashburn, P. M., *op. cit.*, pp. 3-4.
[58] Gross, *19th Century Physicians*, p. 206.
[59] Francis Papers, New York Public Library.
[60] Gansevoort Papers, New York Public Library. For material in these papers, I am indebted to Miss Mabel Weeks of the Manuscript Division.

This list does not include the many physicians who were members of state legislatures, mayors of towns or authors of popular books, such as David Ramsay and Daniel Drake. Yet all the men named were connected with the political or literary life of the country and as such would have been outstanding. It shows, negatively, that being a doctor was not a handicap. Although medicine had been practiced in colonial times by the clergy, and was a profession of good repute, the unsavory stories of grave-robbing by medical students and the quarrels in the medical schools must have detracted somewhat from its prestige. Medical discoveries were not sufficiently spectacular to gain public attention. And, therefore, the profession suffered, as we shall see later, in the repeal of existing laws or the failure to pass new laws protecting its practice.

In this discussion the social position of the medical fraternity has been defined from a limited point of view. Regarded in larger social aspects as a group closely related to the daily lives of people, the profession played an important rôle. After all, the practitioner was present when birth and death were imminent and his ministrations brought him into intimate association with those whom he served. He came, by horseback or by horse and buggy, to answer the call of the sick and distressed. Whatever we may think of his methods, they were the only reputable methods. Perhaps the general population did not view the doctor with such awe as later generations did, but it could not fail to appreciate his fine sense of duty and the intimacy of its relationship with him. We see this part which the doctor played in the following description of a day in the life of John C. Warren, given by his son:

He rose in the winter and breakfasted by candlelight, and went out directly to visit his patients, until one o'clock, when he received patients at his house, until two. He devoted about ten minutes to his dinner; but after this meal, he rested for an hour or more. In the latter part of the afternoon, he visited such patients as required a second visit, took tea at seven; after which he wrote and worked upon the subjects [of interest to him] often until two o'clock, A. M.[61]

[61] Gross, *19th Century Physicians*, pp. 807-808.

CHAPTER VI

Medical Literature

PROFESSIONAL morale can be strengthened by the expression and dissemination of ideas in books, magazines and the publications of societies. Among the writers are systematic thinkers who, by revamping old ideas or by formulating new ones influence the practices of their profession. Their contentions often appear in the standard reference volumes. For those people who do not wish to read at length, the magazines supply articles with briefer statements of theories. But some members of the profession can be reached only through organized societies wherein practices may be discussed with reference to new evidence. Since these societies satisfy the normal craving for association with like-minded individuals they are a potent factor in developing professional attitudes. This chapter treats of the first two factors, books and magazines.

We have seen that few medical works were published in colonial times and in the years following the Revolution. There is evidence of this fact in the obvious joy with which magazine editors welcomed the appearance of new books. When Benjamin Smith Barton brought out his *Collection for an Essay towards a Materia Medica of the United States,* in 1798, the *American Medical Repository* in its review self-consciously ushered in an era in which America would not have to turn to foreigners for a knowledge of its own products.[1] In 1825, the *New York Medical and Physical Journal,* in a similar vein, expressed great satisfac-

---

[1] *Medical Repository,* II, 1798, p. 70.

tion over Dewees's *System of Midwifery*.[2] But, ten years later, the *Boston Medical and Surgical Journal* bemoaned the lack of American authors.[3] Such conflicting opinions resulted from differences in point of view. To those who wanted the United States to be independent of Europe for its medical work's progress seemed disappointingly slow; for others who looked back to colonial days, the writings of American physicians constituted an impressive list. There is no doubt that American books on medical theory and practice increased in quantity and improved in quality as the years passed.

Publications of the period included the proceedings of the medical societies, the medical theses and introductory and valedictory lectures in colleges, certain systematic works which were usually textbooks, and works designed for popular consumption. The first society to publish was the Medical Society of New Haven County, Connecticut, which issued in 1787 *Cases and Observations* in the preface of which the society expressed its willingness to receive and include any scientific communications from physicians outside the county.[4] More important were the *Medical Papers, Communicated to the Massachusetts Medical Society. To which are Subjoined Extracts from various Authors, containing some of the Improvements which have lately been made in Physic and Surgery*, published in 1790, with the hope that they might " produce happy effects, in promoting among ourselves, the improvements of medicine and science of the greatest importance to the public, but which unhappily

---

[2] *New York Medical and Physical Journal* (9 volumes, New York, 1822-1830), IV, 1825, p. 378.

[3] *Boston Medical and Surgical Journal*, XIII, 1835, p. 33.

[4] Medical Society of New-Haven, *Cases and Observations* (New Haven, 1788), Preface.

in this country, has hitherto been too little cultivated." [5] Gradually other societies followed Massachusett's example, and at the end of the period every medical society published its transactions, even though the volumes were but five or six pages. The leading societies such as Massachusetts, New York, Connecticut and New Jersey eventually had volumes containing case histories and accurate accounts of their meetings. Some of them used the transactions to give the profession valuable reference works, as when the Massachusetts Medical Society published fifteen volumes of the *Library of Practical Medicine* which consisted chiefly of Copeland's *Medical Dictionary*.[6] Probably the finest work which the medical societies produced was the *United States Pharmacopœia*, published in 1820 as a result of a meeting in Washington of delegates from the medical societies.

The theses of the students and the lectures of the professors require only passing notice. Theses, at the beginning of the period, were written in Latin and were published. As time passed, however, both requirements seem to have been dropped. Poorly written, they were seldom contributions of importance. Samuel Gross, writing on medical literature in 1876, gives the opinion of one who, as professor in various medical schools, had to correct such works:

Of this variety of medical literature our colleges have huge piles, for every spring, in the Ides of March, large additions are made to their archives, usually badly written, not infrequently ungrammatical, generally devoid of scientific information, and of no use to anybody, for it is not too much to say that not one in fifty affords the slightest evidence of competency, proficiency, or ability in the candidates for graduation. Often, indeed, they are not even composed by him.[7]

[5] Clarke *et al., American Medicine, 1776-1876*, p. 50; Massachusetts Medical Society, *Medical Papers*, 1790, Pref. iii.

[6] Massachusetts Medical Society, *Medical Papers*, VII, 1845, p. 86.

[7] Gross, *American Medical Literature* (Phila., 1876), pp. 55-57.

The introductory lectures may not have been ungrammatical, but they were verbose and usually designed to impress the student by eloquence and Latin quotations, rather than by their scientific knowledge.[8]

American authors of books on medicine and surgery have already been discussed in the chapter dealing with education and textbooks. Benjamin Rush was the outstanding author with his five volumes on *Medical Observations and Inquiries* published in 1788 and 1789 and two subsequent volumes in 1807 and 1812. Caspar Wistar and William E. Horner published in anatomy; John Dorsey and Philip Syng Physick were our authorities on surgery, although Valentine Mott's edition of Velpeau was largely his own work. The writings of Dewees, Eberle and Meigs on midwifery were genuine contributions of skillful practitioners. Scotsman, though Dunglison was, his diverse and authoritative writings after his arrival in this country in 1824 were credited to the American profession. On medical jurisprudence, T. R. Beck's work was as praiseworthy as that of Benjamin Silliman on the subject of chemistry. J. Murray and Nathaniel Chapman advanced the study of materia medica. Other writers, among a fairly large number worthy of mention, were Samuel Bard, Barton, Bigelow, Webster, John Redman Coxe, John C. Warren and George B. Wood, the last of whom writing at the end of the period, produced his noteworthy *Treatise on the Practice of Medicine*.[9]

[8] A. M. A. Transactions, 1848, pp. 249-289; my own impression after looking through a large number of these addresses is a series of short sentences and exclamation marks.

[9] *Cf. supra*, Chapter III; an excellent account and criticism of American medical literature is in Gross's work of the same title issued in Philadelphia in 1876. Gross graduated from the University of Pennsylvania Medical School about 1824 and as a student of medicine, after graduation, and as a teacher studied broadly and was well qualified to look back in the centennial year and evaluate medical writing.

All of these men lived north of the Mason-Dixon Line, and a large number practiced in Philadelphia. This city was so well represented because it was the cultural center of the colonies as well as the home of the first medical college. Larger than New York, until 1830, it was less torn by petty quarrels and produced the finest physicians of the period. We may accept the explanation for the lack of southern writing offered by Richard Arnold when he said:

I wish there was more industry at the South among medical men. Yet it must be recollected that the situation of Medical men at the South and in one of the large cities at the North, where the *writing* men reside, is very different. There a man waits for 10 years to get into practice. He has time and the splendid medical libraries afford him material to dilate to the utmost on the practice he obtains. Here, practice engrosses almost all the attention, and cut off from books, comparatively, there is not that incentive to write here as at the North. However, the experience of the Southern Physicians would afford excellent materials worthy of a permanent record.[10]

But North or South it is true that much of the work of American medical writers consisted in editing works of British authors, a fact admitted by the American Medical Association in its report of 1848.[11]

This editing seems to have been done under contract, for John W. Francis received $500 for his edition of Denman's *Midwifery* with the promise of $200 for each successive edition.[12] Since copyright laws did not have much international authority, many works by prominent Europeans were pirated. Francis explained to R. Thomas, author of

[10] Arnold, *Letters*, pp. 18-19.

[11] A. M. A. *Transactions*, 1848, p. 286.

[12] Francis Letters, in New York Public Library. In a letter to Mrs. G. Bliss dated April 18, 1821.

The Modern Practice of Physic, that neither he nor Thomas's editor, Hosack, but the booksellers had cheated him out of several thousand dollars due on his popular work (which seems to have been published on a royalty basis).[13] With regard to publication of American works, the author sent his book to several publishers, hoping that some one of them might buy the copyright. In this manner, John D. Godman wrote Messrs. H. C. Carey and Lea of Philadelphia, prominent medical publishers, "to dispose of the copyright" on his book.[14] Once these matters were settled, the author sent his book to the magazines for "notice" or review.

Still another type of medical literature was designed for the public. To distinguish between the work of professional men and charlatans in the field of such publication is not always easy. In these books the filtration of ideas from one generation to the next is very clear. The long prescriptions of the eighteenth century live again in the works of many "popular" writers who wrote without benefit of medical education. The distinction between the two types is that the regular profession usually limited itself to general advice upon conduct or upon preserving health whereas quacks prescribed treatment for specific diseases.

The most popular subject with the profession was health preservation. Two books, one published at the end of the period and the other shortly after its close, give us an accurate account of professional opinion on this subject. John C. Warren called his volume *The Preservation of Health* and Elizabeth Blackwell, the first woman to graduate from a medical college in the United States, entitled hers the *Laws of Life*. Opinions common to both were that exercise in

[13] *Ibid.,* April 28, 1821.

[14] Gratz Collection, Case 7, Box 29; Gross, *American Medical Literature,* pp. 66-67 points out that Eberle's copyright on his *Materia Medica* sold for $500; he infers that this was accepted practice.

the fresh air, simple foods and avoidance of stimulants, such as alcohol, tea, coffee and tobacco, are essential to good health.[15] Elizabeth Blackwell believed that physical education by delaying puberty in young boys would ward off licentiousness. Warren added that "a great number of young persons, especially of the male sex, lose their health from a vitiated imagination, the prevention and cure of this should be one of the greatest objects of attention to parents and instructors." [16]

William A. Alcott, who preached from 1836 to 1856 the doctrines of self-control, exercise, simple living and Victorian behavior, is outstanding in this field. He stressed in his book on *Tea and Coffee: Their Physical, Intellectual and Moral Effects on the Human System* the danger of these stimulants. In the *Young Wife,* he devotes a chapter to a discussion of Sobriety which begins:

Let not the reader startle, as if he supposed I was going to charge the female sex with the grosser forms of intemperance. . . . Not but that there are individuals among the sex who have sunk thus low—a few, even of those who are dignified with the sacred and responsible name of wife.

He concludes by telling at great length the evils of tea and coffee.[17]

In these books and the *Vegetable Diet,* which he endorsed, and *Lectures on Life and Health* he inculcated the moralities which we associate with that period. He stressed the important position of a wife, her duty to her family, her ability to make or unmake her husband by controlling his nature,

[15] Warren, J. C., *Preservation of Health* (Boston, 1846), pp. 115-119, did say that the sugar and not the tea was harmful.

[16] *Ibid.,* pp. 115-119; Elizabeth Blackwell, *Laws of Life...* (N. Y., 1852), p. 28.

[17] Alcott, William A., *The Young Wife* (Boston, 1838), p. 192.

the necessity of delicacy of language which would not permit a " My stars! " or similar expressions because they " besides being indelicate, savor not a little of profanity. They are exceedingly unbecoming, but especially in females." [18]

These ideas are significant because they had the endorsement of the profession. The belief in the sacredness of women and the desire to protect them from the vulgarities of life led the profession to ignore many topics which we discuss today without demur. Approval of Alcott both by his profession and the public appears in the enthusiastic endorsement which the *Boston Medical and Surgical Journal* gave *The Young Mother,* when it sold out 2000 copies and a second edition of 3000 was announced.[19]

MEDICAL MAGAZINES

The lack of magazines in colonial times and the poor quality of those which were later published illustrate the disorganized state of the medical profession in early America. We have mentioned that articles appeared in the *Columbian Magazine*, the *American Museum* and in the proceedings of both the American Philosophical Society and the American Academy of Arts and Sciences. The first medical magazine was Mitchill's *American Medical Repository,* begun in New York in 1797. Dr. Mitchill was an enthusiastic innovator. Although he took his degree in medicine, he was not a practicing physician, and his many interests from politics to language detracted from whole-hearted promotion of any single enterprise. To us much of the *Repository,* as it was commonly and affectionately called, is amusing and valueless. Historically, however, it is important. It furnished the early American physician with his first regular publication of medical news and information; and, as the

[18] *Ibid.*, p. 82.
[19] *Boston Medical and Surgical Journal*, XIV, 1836, pp. 381-382.

forerunner in a new field, it set an example to the profession. With the success of the *Repository,* medical magazines increased rapidly until by 1850 the number exceeded the need and demand.

During the years from 1797 to 1850 one hundred and seventeen medical journals appeared. Naturally many failed or were merged with more successful competitors, but the number shows the impetus within the profession to spread its ideas. Analysing these publications by decades, we find that from 1800 to 1810, six magazines appeared. These included the *Charleston Medical Register,* edited by David Ramsay in 1803; *The Philadelphia Medical Museum,* edited by John Redman Coxe, which was founded in 1804 and continued until 1811: *The Baltimore Medical and Physical Recorder,* conducted by Tobias Watkins for the two years of its life, 1808 and 1809; and the *New York Medical and Philosophical Journal and Review,* which was published in New York from 1809 to 1811 but evidently could not compete with the more popular *Repository.* These magazines were published only in cities which served a large community.

This type of publication reached New England in the *New England Journal of Medicine and Surgery* of 1812, which, after its merger with the *Boston Medical Intelligencer* in 1828 as the *Boston Medical and Surgical Journal,* was to serve that district for many years. Besides this journal nine others were brought out before 1820. All were published in Philadelphia, New York and Baltimore. From 1820 to 1830, twenty-eight magazines were established; some of these were the more scientific and important of the period. The *Boston Medical and Surgical Journal* has already been mentioned. The *Philadelphia Journal of Medical and Physical Sciences* of 1820 " supported by an association of physicians and edited by N. Chapman " merged in 1828, with the *Philadelphia Monthly Journal of Medicine and Surgery* as the

American Journal of the Medical Sciences, which under the editorship of Chapman and Isaac Hays, was to become one of the foremost medical magazines in the United States. Publication, following the frontier at a discreet distance, crossed the Alleghenies. John D. Godman published the *Western Medical and Physical Journal* at Cincinnati which merged in 1828 with Guy W. Wright's and J. M. Mason's *Ohio Medical Repository of Original and Selected Essays and Intelligence,* founded in 1826, to form the *Western Journal of Medical and Physical Sciences* under the editorship of Daniel Drake. This periodical was discontinued in 1838 but was revived in 1840 and consolidated with the *Louisville Journal of Medicine and Surgery* as the *Western Journal of Medicine and Surgery.* In the South, the *Carolina Journal of Medicine, Science and Agriculture* existed only for one year. New developments were such specialized publications as *The Vaccine Inquirer,* which ran through five numbers in Baltimore from 1822 to 1824, and the *Journal of the Philadelphia College of Pharmacy* founded in 1825 and merged, ten years later, with the *Journal of Pharmacy.*

Of the twenty-nine new magazines listed during the years from 1830 to 1840, only two were noteworthy. The first was the *Baltimore Medical and Surgical Journal and Review,* of 1833, edited by E. Geddings which became the *North American Archives of Medical and Surgical Sciences,* in 1834. The other, *The Eclectic Journal of Medicine* and its partner, the *Select Medical Library,* begun by John Bell in 1836 and continued by him as the *Select Medical Library and Bulletin of Medical Science* until 1846, contained in addition to the usual case studies and news, reprints of valuable published works. Its cost prevented large circulation, and it failed to exert the influence anticipated. The geographical expansion continued with the *Southern Medical and Surgical Journal* and the *Louisville Journal of Medicine and Surgery,* which lasted only two numbers but was later, in 1840, revived and merged with the *Western Journal of the Medical and Physical Sciences* to form the *Western Journal of Medicine and Surgery*. The separation of dentistry from surgery was one of the medical changes of this period. The *American Journal of Dental Science* of 1839, published simultaneously in New York City, Philadelphia, Boston and Baltimore, demonstrated the extent of this separation, for the magazine had sufficient support from those interested in dentistry alone. The *Cholera Gazette* of 1832, a weekly edited by Isaac Hays of Philadelphia, and the *Cholera Bulletin* of the same year put out by an " Association of physicians " three times a week in New York City from July 9th to August 31st of the same year, both exemplify the increased social conscience of the profession. Cholera running through Europe reached America in 1832, and the profession organized as effectively as possible to stop it. These publications were attempts by medical men to reach both the public and physicians with all information.

None of the forty-four magazines, which appeared from 1840 to 1850, had enduring influence. The more specialized magazines, however, showed an increasing scientific spirit. General medical periodicals merely spread into sections hitherto dependent upon the larger cities. It meant that the profession was aware of its increasing strength; and it probably helped the organization of medical societies. Examples of this expansion are the *Buffalo Medical Journal* of 1845 under the editorship of Austin Flint, and the development of a periodical for the region west and north of the Ohio in the *Illinois Medical and Surgical Journal* of 1845, which assumed its sectional aspects in 1848 under the title of the *Northwestern Medical and Surgical Journal*. The Southwest was finally provided with monthly medical news by the *New Orleans Medical and Surgical Journal*, which, after merging with the projected *Louisiana Medical and Surgical Journal* in 1845, became the successful *New Orleans Medical and Surgical Journal.* Likewise, the south Atlantic states had a permanent magazine in the *Southern Journal of Medicine and Pharmacy* edited by J. L. Smith and S. D. Sinkler in 1846 and 1847 and continued by P. C. Gaillard and H. W. DeSaussure as the *Charleston Medical Journal and Review.*

Thus by 1850 all the settled portions of the country had medical publications of varying degrees of value but almost all of them more scientific than the early publications. In the specialized fields the *American Journal of Insanity,* begun in Utica, New York, in 1844 by the medical officers of the New York State Lunatic Asylum as a quarterly study of the progress in mental care, was ably edited and a source of information for reforms in a field practically neglected until 1830. The *American Annals of the Deaf and Dumb,* emanating from Hartford, Connecticut in 1847 satisfied a similar need. *Wood's Quarterly Retrospect of American and Foreign Practical Medicine and Surgery* for the two years from 1847 to 1849 reflects an increasing interest in bibliography. Stockton and Co.'s *Dental Intelligencer* of 1843 with its advertising and scientific studies represents the attempt of a commercial company to advance its products within the profession. Dentistry, itself, by 1847, was able to support one more magazine, the *Dental Register of the West.*

A numerical study of these publications would be misleading without a qualifying discussion of the life of the magazines. An estimate of their duration can be reached by classifying them according to the number of years which they ran and by considering mergers and continuations under new titles as one magazine. Such a simplification reduces the total number to ninety-five journals. Of these nineteen existed less than one year; eight, for only one year; sixteen, for two years; thirteen, for nine to fifteen years; and one, the *Medical Repository*, for twenty-four years with short interruptions. In 1850 twenty-four magazines circulated, of which the *Boston Medical and Surgical Journal* dated from 1812 and the *American Journal of Medical Sciences* from 1825. With these exceptions it is apparent that the average life-expectancy of a medical magazine was short.

With regard to place of publication, New York with twenty-five magazines, Philadelphia with nineteen, Boston and Baltimore with ten each were the centers. Periodicals were published in Charleston, Augusta and New Orleans in the South; five were established at Cincinnati and two at Columbus in Ohio. Other places of publication were Chicago, Indianapolis, St. Louis, Louisville, Lexington, Buffalo, Albany, Utica and Hartford. Publication of the same magazine in various cities was not common. The only examples were in Lexington and Cincinnati, Cincinnati and Louisville; the *United States Medical and Surgical Journal* was published in New York and Philadelphia; the *American Journal of Dental Sciences* was issued in New York, Philadelphia, Boston and Baltimore; and the *Transylvania Medical Journal* was published in Lexington and Louisville. The whole country was thus furnished with medical journals. Since they differed in merit rather than in organization, it is possible to study them as a group.

The methods of editing were three. In some cases a physician acting as editor took command for a publisher and selected the materials from contributions. At other times associations of physicians were formed with general charge of acceptance and arrangement of material. Thus the *New England Journal of Medicine and Surgery* printed the following notice in 1824:

The *New-England Journal of Medicine and Surgery* will in future be conducted by the subscribers who have previously formed part of the Association, by which it has hitherto been supported. The other gentlemen of the Association have relinquished all share in its management, and are to be considered as entirely free from any responsibility with regard to the manner in which it shall be conducted. The present Editors, however, have reason to believe, that as individuals, they will still continue to manifest an interest in its success, and contribute by their labours to its reputation and usefulness.[20]

Still another type of publication was the *Transylvania Medical Journal,* which was published by the faculty of the Transylvania Medical College. To follow the changes which took place in the editorial departments of these journals would lead one into a confusion of names.

Contributions of articles and news seem to have been voluntary. There was some effort to get reports on certain conditions, particularly the attempts of Samuel Latham Mitchill to survey local diseases and climatic conditions. The single evidence of remuneration for these articles is a statement by Samuel Gross in 1876 that the journals paid one dollar a page, which may have been an innovation after 1850.[21] A departure from this method of relying upon voluntary contributions and extracts from other magazines was a large list of collaborators in the *American Journal of Medical Sciences,* which, included Jacob Bigelow of Harvard, Nathaniel Chapman of the University of Pennsylvania, W. E. Daniel of Savannah, J. B. Davidge of the University of Maryland, S. H. Dickson of the Medical College of South Carolina, Thomas Fearn of Alabama, David Hosack of Rutgers Medical College and New York City and Thomas Sewall of the Columbian Medical College of Washington. Another innovation by this magazine was its announcement in 1828 that henceforth it would not accept anonymous con-

---

[20] *New England Journal of Medicine and Surgery,* XIII, p. 336.
[21] Gross, *American Medical Literature,* pp. 66-67.

tributions.[22] As many magazines as could afford it made arrangements with European doctors for reprints. The *Philadelphia Journal of Medical and Physical Sciences* announced in 1825 that arrangements had been made to get the medical and scientific journals of France, Germany, Italy and other countries as well as their new medical works.[23]

It was frequently charged that editors used their magazines to foster their own medical opinions. The New York *Dissector* pointed out, on its cover, that it was a "novel experiment of a perfectly independent Medical Journal" and that its great success (in the editor's opinion, for it soon disappeared) was due to this fact.[24] Again so respectable a weekly as the *Boston Medical Intelligencer* protested in 1825: "We are perfectly independent and neither care for the frowns of those who dislike us, nor the envy of those who make themselves miserable in railing against our manner of writing medical reports." [25] Undoubtedly this quarreling helps to explain the rise and fall of editors and publications and accounts for the fact that New York City was without any medical journal in the year 1837.[26]

The high cost of publication made it difficult for journals to support themselves. The *Boston Medical and Surgical Journal,* in 1836, exclaimed: "There is not a profitable Medical Journal in this country and what is still more surprising, there never was one—and worse still, there is not likely to be one." [27] The subscription rates, which were to pay expenses, ran from one dollar and fifty cents to five dollars. The *New York Medical and Philosophical Journal* of 1809

[22] *American Journal of Medical Sciences,* IV, Notice.
[23] *Philadelphia Journal of Medical and Physical Sciences,* XI, Notice.
[24] *The New York Dissector,* III (New York, 1846), Notice.
[25] *Boston Medical Intelligencer,* III, p. 67.
[26] *Boston Medical and Surgical Journal,* XVI, 1837, p. 305.
[27] *Ibid.,* XV, 1836, p. 240.

sold for seventy-five cents a copy, one dollar and fifty cents a year.[28] The *Boston Medical and Surgical Journal* sold for two dollars a year at the beginning of its publication. The *Philadelphia Medical and Physical Journal* sold for five dollars in 1824.[29] The *Baltimore Philosophical Journal and Review* was unsuccessful at five dollars per year.[30] The *American Journal of Dental Science* cost three dollars per year.[31] The prices of this magazine and the *Illinois and Indiana Medical and Surgical Journal* at two dollars per year are representative rates.[32]

Advertising, which was run on the covers, was the other source of income. As a survey of the journals will show, this was not large. In 1843 the *Boston Medical and Surgical Journal*, a weekly publication so large that it was then issued in two volumes a year, wrote:

As the present plan of a distinct advertising sheet will probably accommodate all who may in future wish to avail themselves of it, we hope to meet the expectations of all. It may be understood, therefore, in future, that the advertisements of publishers, booksellers, druggists, instrument makers, importers, medical schools, hospitals, societies, and all other medical notices, can have ready attention, and be allowed to remain in type according to the directions of those who order them.[33]

The foregoing quotation not only gives the amount of space allotted but the type of advertising as well. Evidently "all other medical notices" was a term covering many

[28] *New York Medical and Philosophical Journal and Review*, I, Flyleaf.
[29] *Philadelphia Journal of Medical and Physical Sciences*, IX, Cover.
[30] *Baltimore Philosophical Journal and Review*, I, 1823, Cover.
[31] *American Journal of Dental Science* (10 volumes, N. Y., Balt., Bost. and Phila., 1839-1850), I, p. 7.
[32] *The Illinois and Indiana Medical and Surgical Journal* (2 volumes, Chicago and Indianapolis, 1846-1848), I, cover.
[33] *Boston Medical and Surgical Journal*, XXVIII, 1843, p. 23.

types, for the report on Medical Literature by the committee of the American Medical Association in 1848 stated:

> The advertising portion of the journals seems to be considered by some editors as beyond the jurisdiction of medical ethics. It is to this opinion, or more probably to mere inadvertence, that the physician owes the privilege of reading before he opens one of the prominent journals, the notice of one Dr. Beach's Medical Works, for which he has received numerous gold medals from the various crowned heads of Europe, and diplomas from the most learned colleges in the Old World.[34]

The fact that the publisher often controlled publication and that magazines constantly needed money may have driven many editors to accept such advertising. The rates of the *American Journal of Medical Sciences* for 1838 certainly were not exorbitant, with one page at six dollars per issue and any fraction of a page at three dollars.[35]

The contents of the magazines depict the interests of the profession. The table of contents usually was: first, reports or case studies under the heading "original communications"; second, "selections" or reprints from other magazines here and abroad; third, reviews of recent publications; and fourth, general news, which included items from medical colleges and medical societies, excerpts from other periodicals, occasional editorials and mere literary chit-chat.

Scientific discoveries of interest to the profession were not sufficiently numerous to supply monthly magazines with news. The aims of the magazines were summarized by the *Medical Repository* in 1803:

> Our leading objects since the first establishment of this work uniformly have been, to form a centre of communication for the contributors to science in all parts of the United States;

[34] A. M. A. *Transactions*, 1848, p. 284. Report on medical literature.
[35] *American Journal of Medical Sciences*, XXII, 1838, p. 259.

to rescue from oblivion the fruits of the experience and observation of medical brethren, . . . to allure men of talents from the inactivity which diffidence and retirement are too apt to impose, by soliciting their communications, to give early and authentic information of all such discoveries and improvement in every part of the civilized world as fall within the limits assigned to our publication, to offer some small return to the learned nations of Europe for the obligations we owe them, our original instructors and parents in science; and, finally, to institute a national work which may assist similar designs elsewhere in exciting the energies, developing the productions, and hastening the maturity of a young and rising empire. How far we have succeeded in these endeavors, is willingly submitted to the candour and justice of the public.[86]

Whether or not the *Medical Repository* achieved all these ends, it certainly helped the development of American medical journalism and, as we shall see presently, European writers borrowed from it and from subsequent medical journals.

The pages of the journals were filled with descriptions of prevalent diseases. The *Medical Repository* spent much space contending that the origin of yellow fever was local. Its twenty-first volume contained a series of papers on the " summer epidemic of Yellow-Fever " in North America and the West Indies. Volume eighteen contained a systematic study of the " Winter Epidemic " of 1812-1813-1814- and 1815. Yet the space, which in earlier volumes was filled by Priestly's defense of the outworn theory of phlogiston against the attacks of Waterhouse, who upheld the point of view of Lavoisier, was later taken by an argument between Dr. Ives and Dr. Chatard over the use of ergot in labor. In other words, the medical magazine (and the profession) was more interested in new discoveries than in theories of doubtful validity. It was in the publicity which the magazines

[86] *Medical Repository*, VI, p. ix.

gave to discoveries, such as that which the *Boston Medical and Surgical Journal* accorded anesthesia, that positive aid was given to scientific advancement. Because these discoveries appeared in such a medium, they reached a greater number of physicians than if they had been published in more expensive works. Whenever the journals promulgated new methods and theories, they performed a service which far over-balanced their retailing of midwive's tales.

In furthering general scientific principles the periodicals accomplished more than might be expected. They constantly emphasized the need for dissection and a knowledge of anatomy.[37] They attacked adulteration of drugs.[38] Here and there voices were lifted condemning the over-use of drugs and the usual methods of treating disease. In this vein, the *Boston Medical Intelligencer*, in 1826, wrote that, " by diet and regime, for example, more may be done for the dyspeptic than by calomel, bark, or brandy." [39] The advocacy of a better diet was partly reaction to the inadequacies of the old methods and also to the success of the quack. It was carried further in the health journals, in which Graham eventually was immortalized in the name of a cracker. In these journals and in many others during the 1840's, there was a growing demand for physical education. In the *Journal of Health and Monthly Miscellany*, Walter Channing, a well-known Boston physician, ran four articles on this essential of a healthy life.[40]

The periodicals also promoted improvement in professional standards by discussing medical education, by attacking

[37] *New York Medical and Philosophical Journal*, II, p. 67 for example.

[38] *Medical Repository*, II, 1798, pp. 224-225 contains an article by John MacLean, Professor of Chemistry in the College of New Jersey, on the *Nature of Septic Gases* and an article in the *American Journal of Pharmacy*, I, pp. 11-13.

[39] *Boston Medical Intelligencer*, IV, pp. 54-55.

[40] *Journal of Health and Monthly Miscellany* (Boston, 1847), pp. 170-172, 193-197, 224-230, 295-299.

quackery and by advocating adequate organization and legal protection. Regularly they printed whatever news the colleges made available to them. Although the local journals confined their comments to the work of schools in their immediate vicinity, the more important magazines made special efforts to survey the whole field of medical education. They watched with considerable attention the work of quacks and discussed them in many articles. They conducted frequent surveys to show the comparative status of the profession in various districts with regard to numbers, fees and educational facilities. This activity stirred the profession, and it is noteworthy that the magazines, even more than the colleges, were instrumental in fostering the medical convention which led to the formation of the American Medical Association.

Besides purely professional advancement the journals aided causes which they deemed worthy. For example, they supported the temperance movement. The *Repository* made a study of saloons in New York, and, closely related to the saloons, the conditions of workingmen. Even the bawdy houses were subjected to examination. These studies and others, such as the survey of the water conditions of New York and Philadelphia, not only seem appropriate in a magazine entitled " repository " but were considered proper subjects for a medical journal.[41]

Reviews of recent books which appeared in the journals frequently reflected personal prejudice. Although the reviews of the *American Journal of Medical Sciences* were the most impartial, treatment of an author usually depended upon the personal attitude of the editors. We have the point of view of an author in a letter from Charles Caldwell to a friend in Philadelphia in which he said,

[41] *Medical Repository*, VII, p. 89; VI, pp. 333-34; VII, pp. 90-91; III, p. 65.

permit me to ask your acceptance of a copy of my late Indiana address of which I send you two. The other you may give, if you think proper, to some one of the Editors of your city, and let him notice, *if* he please . . . As a writer I ask no favours; and from the Philadelphia press I have no reason to expect any. It has never been friendly to me—but the *reverse*—I have never bowed to it, now in any way flattered it—and never will. Other *presses in this* and other lands have done me justice— and that is enough.[42]

Reviews could be caustic, varying greatly with the personal feelings of the reviewers. In the course of a twenty-five-page criticism of David Hosack's fifty-one page monograph on *Febrile Contagion,* the *Medical Repository* said,

We will now take leave of this academic nondescript and its author, in the hope that when we next hear from him, if it be not on a subject more interesting, it will at least be in a manner less offensive; for if anything can exceed the mortification of being obliged to write these remarks, it is the conviction we feel that they are but too well merited.[43]

Regarding the same book, the *Philadelphia Journal of Medical and Physical Science* could say that, while differing with Hosack in his views on the origin of yellow fever, they would always applaud his "talent, industry, and success" in investigating the subject and especially his discovery of immunity after one attack.[44] Hosack at that time, 1820, was a professor in the College of Physicians and Surgeons and six years later was to lead the faculty away to found Rutgers Medical College. He was too active a man to remain outside the professional quarreling prevalent in New York City

---

[42] Dreer Collection, Pennsylvania Historical Society, I, Letter dated October 24, 1836.

[43] *Medical Repository,* XXI, 1821, p. 229.

[44] *Philadelphia Journal of Medical and Physical Sciences,* I, 1820, p. 443.

at that time; and he was too successful a man to be free from the envy of his professional brethren. If the *Repository* did not find sufficient reason in Hosack himself for its criticism, it did in his point of view on the origin of yellow fever which disagreed with the commonly accepted local-origin theory.

Most reviews reflected the vanity and verbosity of the author and contained little genuine criticism. The subscribers to the journals did not receive a comprehensive survey of medical publication. Often the editors turned aside from the medical field to notice books of little medical interest. Occasionally, these digressions should have been helpful, especially when the *New York Medical and Physical Journal and Review* discussed *An English Grammar: comprehending the Principles and Rules of the Language*.[45]

Relations among the editors of the magazines were more cordial than the relations between reviewers and authors. Lesser journals were inclined to be hypercritical, as when the *American Medical Recorder* disparaged the somewhat loud patriotism of the *Philadelphia Journal of Medical and Physical Science*.[46] If a fly-by-night publication appeared, the older editors might take it to task. The *Boston Medical Intelligencer,* for example, admonished the *Æsculapian* to which the latter replied by pointing to its success without the aid of the well established magazines. But twenty-six issues later the new journal wound up its affairs because there was too much competition and people did not pay their subscriptions.[47]

Larger journals, however, could afford a more generous spirit. In 1810, the *New York Medical and Physical Journal and Review* extended greetings to a new publication

[45] *New York Medical and Philosophical Journal*, II, pp. 272-273.
[46] *The American Medical Recorder*, IV, pp. 169-208.
[47] *Æsculapian Register* (Phila., 1824), I, pp. 44-45, 198.

in that city with the statement that the more publications the better preservation of facts.⁴⁸ In 1825 the *Philadelphia Journal of Medical and Physical Sciences* welcomed the *North American Medical and Surgical Journal*,⁴⁹ and two years later the *Boston Medical Intelligencer* praised the same magazine liberally in an editorial.⁵⁰ As late as 1840 the *Boston Medical and Surgical Journal* announced the *Homeopathic Examiner* with a statement that it hoped to receive the magazine regularly in order to transcribe to its own pages whatever might be of " utility to the profession at large." ⁵¹

Whatever minor dissensions appeared among the journals they all joined in the prevalent nationalism. The cultural dependence of America upon England proved irksome and at times led to extravagant statements. It was this spirit which caused the *Philadelphia Journal of Medical and Physical Sciences* to run as its foreword the classic of British snobbery from the *Edinburgh Review*: " In the four quarters of the globe, who reads an American book? or goes to an American play? or looks at an American picture or statue? *What does the world yet owe to American Physicians and Surgeons?* " ⁵² The *Medical Repository*, despite an acknowledgment of our indebtedness to Europe, started this self conscious nationalism. At times it took a bombastic vein as it did in the prospectus of the *Emporium of Arts and Sciences,* which stated:

It is remarkable that notwithstanding the scattered state of our population, our citizens are better informed and have fewer prejudices than any people upon the globe. Liberty, the surest

⁴⁸ *New York Medical and Physical Journal*, II, p. 285.

⁴⁹ *Philadelphia Journal of Medical and Physical Sciences*, XI, pp. 416-417.

⁵⁰ *Boston Medical Intelligencer*, V, p. 391.

⁵¹ *Boston Medical and Surgical Journal*, XXII, p. 82.

⁵² *Philadelphia Journal of Medical and Physical Sciences*, I, Cover.

pledge of free inquiry, is one prime source of the advantages we enjoy. Unfettered in our press—unshackled in our conscience, man here possesses means of happiness as perfect as is consistent with his nature.[53]

At other times journals basked in the light of foreign praise. For instance, the *Medical Repository* quoted an English physician as saying, that, with the exception of vaccination, America had done more than any other country to advance medicine. The *Repository* went on to suggest that British publications credit Americans with articles taken from our magazines.[54] In 1829, the *American Journal of Medical Sciences* noted with justifiable pride that Professor Jackson's "Case of Mercurial Irritation," which first appeared in its pages, had been copied in two European journals, and that two other articles had been extensively transcribed throughout Europe.[55] Petty chauvinism, on the other hand, characterized the objection of the *Philadelphia Journal of Medical and Physical Sciences* to the appointment of an Englishman instead of an American to the Virginia Institute of Medicine.[56] And in 1831, the *Boston Medical and Surgical Journal* became positively indignant when the *Lancet*, an English publication, suggested, certainly with some truth, that impoverished English doctors emigrated to America.[57] This nationalistic spirit was inevitable when American medicine had so little to give the world; as the profession improved and contributed to universal knowledge, such bombast diminished.

[53] *Emporium of Arts and Sciences* (2 volumes, Phila., 1812-1813), I, Cover.
[54] *Medical Repository*, XI, Pref. iv-v.
[55] *American Journal of Medical Sciences*, V, p. 8.
[56] *Philadelphia Journal of Medical and Physical Sciences*, IX, pp. 400-409.
[57] *Boston Medical and Surgical Journal*, III, pp. 115-116.

It is apparent, that, throughout this period, medical magazines left much to be desired, but with the passage of time many absurdities disappeared. There was a decided change from the *Medical Repository* with its dissertations on *Manures* and whatever, for the moment, interested S. L. Mitchill, to later magazines such as the *American Journal of Medical Sciences* in the general field of medicine and the *American Journal of Insanity*, the *Dental News Letter* or the *Medical and Surgical Register* with their specialized accounts. When the *Boston Journal of Philosophy and the Arts* expired in 1830, the old-style medical periodical which relied upon an association with other sciences disappeared from the eastern section of the country. As the cultural frontier spread West, the early connection between medicine and other subjects was repeated, but the magazines of the frontier or semi-frontier regions never became quite so discursive as the early journals. The imagination of Mitchill with his suggestion of *Fredon* as the name for *America;* " *Fredonian* a sonorous name " for citizens; *Frede* as a short name; *Fredish* as an adjective, was never duplicated.[58] Nor was it necessary to publish a recipe for beer under the caption " To LOVERS OF GOOD BEER " or note the invention of an onion-planting machine.[59] More first-rate magazines were available to medical students in 1850 than the three, the *American Journal of Medical Sciences, the North American Medical and Surgical Journal,* and the *New England Journal of Medicine and Surgery,* which were recommended by the Massachusetts Medical Society in 1832.[60]

Thus with all their faults of meager knowledge, reprinting, personal feuds, petty reviewing and nationalism, the periodicals did improve. The harshest criticism came from

[58] *Medical Repository*, VI, p. 449.
[59] *Boston Medical Intelligencer*, IV, pp. 334.
[60] Massachusetts Medical Society, *Medical Papers*, V, 1832, pp. 71-79.

the American Medical Association in 1848, in the following words.

The proportion allotted to these several divisions varies very much. Taking into consideration the usual difference of type in the original and borrowed matter and the very liberal extracts which the reviewers commonly make from the work before them, it will be found that a very large part of all the journals is made up of quotations and to a considerable extent of the same quotations, whatever may be the particular journal examined. The committee have been struck with the fact, that the same articles have been presented over and over again to the notice, in many different periodicals, each borrowing from its neighbours the best papers of the last preceding number, so that the perusal of many is not so much more laborious than that of a single one, as would be anticipated. The ring of editors sit in each other's laps, with perfect propriety, and great convenience it is true, but with a wonderful saving in the article of furniture.[61]

[61] A. M. A. *Transactions*, 1848, p. 256.

CHAPTER VII

MEDICAL REGULATIONS AND SOCIETIES

WHILE the medical profession was developing its professional spirit in its schools and literature, it was also organizing medical societies. At the same time, the people and their legislators were becoming more aware of the social importance of medicine and public health; indeed, the two developments are parallel. In this chapter, we shall examine some of the irregular systems which challenged the allopath, trace the rise and decline of regulatory laws and finally discuss the history and activities of the medical societies.

IRREGULAR MEDICINE

Probably no profession has been so harassed by pretenders as the medical profession. From early times to the present, harmful and harmless systems of quackery have risen, only to die and then to be revived again under some new name. The end of the eighteenth century witnessed the rise and popularity of the magnetic implement. Although many were developed, the most famous was the Patent Metallic Tractor invented by Elisha Perkins of Connecticut. This Tractor consisted of "two rods of brass and iron, about three inches long, rounded at one end and pointed at the other. One side was half round and the other was flat." These were applied to the afflicted part of the body with a downward stroking movement. In cases of stubborn resistance to the cure they were applied with force sufficient to draw out the inflammation. The Tractors were endorsed by many famous people, brought Perkins a small fortune and made his son wealthy.[1]

The quackery, however, which received most attention during these years was that developed and patented by one Samuel Thomson. The system combined the use of steam and certain vegetable compounds from which the practitioners received the names of " Steam-doctors " and " Botanics." Samuel Thomson, the founder, was born at Alstead, New Hampshire in 1769. When his child was ill with canker and rash, the regular doctor said that both eyes would be lost. Thomson, by his own account, steamed the child every two hours for a week, applied cold wet cloths to her eyes and finally removed the canker with a wash of rosemary, thereby saving one eye. His discovery of the value of steam and the emetic powers of lobelia leaves was his fortune. The unsuccessful attempt to convict him of witchcraft in 1808 probably won him adherents and sympathy. Benjamin Waterhouse endorsed him, and Rush and Barton of Philadelphia were sympathetic. Finally in 1813, he patented his system, only to become involved in quarrels which necessitated a second patent in 1821. He attracted many followers who bickered and dissented but who brought him and his system a national reputation.[2]

According to his patent, Thomson administered lobelia powder and pulverized cayenne or real pepper to cleanse the stomach, warm up the patient and increase perspiration. A compound of such herbs as marsh rosemary and sumach bark, served as a tea, was sometimes substituted for lobelia leaves and pepper. The bilious condition was corrected by a prescription which called for bitter herb or balmony, poplar

[1] Fishbein, Morris, *Medical Follies* (New York, 1925), pp. 18-19. Gives a clear story of fakes of the past and a fine analysis of their rise and decline; Perkins, B. D., *The Efficacy of Perkins Patent Medicine Tractors* . . . (n. p., n. d.), *passim.*

[2] Thomson, Samuel, *New Guide to Health*; ... (Boston, 1825), *passim.*

bark, wine or spirits and hot water. Once the system was cleansed, a " syrop " of peach kernels or cherry stones, gum myrrh, hot water, two ounces of sugar and a half pint of brandy had a tonic effect.[3] The heating effects of pepper and emetics were supplemented by steam baths. The whole system relied upon harmless herbs and as such may easily have provided salutary competition for the regulars and their somewhat harmful drugs.

The followers of Thomson organized societies and schools. In 1833 the first national convention of Thomsonians was held at Columbus, Ohio, and after subsequent meetings the first national Thomsonian Society was formed in 1840.[4] The practitioners established medical colleges in Georgia, Alabama and Ohio. In addition to these colleges they developed their own medical magazines, one of which ran as its motto Jefferson's statement: " Not only a Reformation in Medicine is necessary but a Revolution." [5]

Thomson, however, was only one of the many pretenders who attacked the practices of the regular physicians and competed with them for patients. In 1836 the *Boston Medical and Surgical Journal* listed the types of doctors as follows: regular, irregular, Broussaisians, Sangradorian, Morrisonian, botanic, regular botanic, Thomsonians, reformed Thomsonian, magnetical, electrical, homeopathic, rootist, herbist, florist and quack.[6] Add to this group the phrenologists and mesmerizers and a fairly complete picture is obtained of the types of medical practitioners at that time.

Besides quack doctors the markets were flooded with books which pretended to cure, as is aways the case, those diseases which baffled regular practices. Or, the writers preyed upon

[3] *New York Medical and Physical Journal*, IX, N. S. I, pp. 211-215.
[4] Wilder, A., *History of Medicine* (New Sharon, Maine, 1901), *passim*.
[5] *Rhode Island Medical Reformer* (Providence, 1843), I, Cover.
[6] *Boston Medical and Surgical Journal*, XV, pp. 241-242.

those who wished to conceal and cure venereal diseases. An example of this type of literature is the compendious volume entitled *The Treasure of Health or a wonderful collection of the most valuable secrets of Medicine; For the cure of all Diseases, Wounds and other accidents . . . also the best Preservation against the Plague, Pestilential Fevers, Small Pox, and other Kinds of Contagious Diseases. Carefully collected by a benevolent Society in Europe. Translated by Lewis Merlin and published in Philadelphia in 1819.*[7]

While the doctor had to contend with irregular practitioners and the books of other pretenders, he faced further competition from the patent medicine industry. Upon "balsams", "panaceas" and "catholicons", the firms of New York City alone were spending "upwards of one hundred thousand dollars annually in advertising."[8] In 1827 the Medical Society of the County of New York investigated such popular medicines as Columbian Syrup, Parker's Vegetable Panacea and Potters' Catholicon, which were designed to cure syphilis, mercurial diseases, scrofula, scurvy, rheumatism, hepatic derangements and chronic eruptions. It was found that they consisted chiefly of concentrated decoctions of sarsaparilla with other ingredients according to the fancy of the manufacturer. In the case of Swaim's Panacea the prescription of Dr. N. J. Quackenboss of New York City had been patented by a bookbinder.[9] The patent medicine venders also dispensed, in pre-Comstockian days, information on contraception and abortion. Female pills were even advertised in the religious press.[10]

[7] *The Treasure of Health* . . . (Phila., 1819). Loaned to the author by Richard McFeeley.

[8] Shryock, Richard H., " Public Relations of the Medical Profession in Great Britain and the United States: 1600-1870." Reprint from *Annals of Medical History*, II, no. 3, of new series, pp. 308-339, p. 316.

[9] *Report of the Medical Society of the City of New York on Nostrums, or Secret Medicines*, Part I (New York, 1827), pp. 29-30, 35.

[10] Shryock, *op. cit.*, p. 316.

THE REGULATION OF THE PRACTICE OF PHYSICK

With such a state of affairs, it is not surprising that laws were passed to limit medical practice to regular physicians. Unfortunately, the profession did not rise to the demands of the public (actually it was never given a fair chance), and the laws were later repealed.

There had been regulation of the medical profession long before the question of licensing practitioners commanded attention. Massachusetts' law of 1649 is usually accepted as the first regulatory act. Previous to this act, however, Virginia had two laws, the first, passed in 1639, of which we learn in the preamble to the act of 1646:

> WHEREAS by the 9th act of the Assembly held the 21st of October, 1639, consideration being had and taken of the imoderate and excessive rates and prices exacted by practitioners in physic and chyrurgery and the complaints made to the then Assembly of the bad consequences thereof. It so happening through the said intollerable exactions that the hearts of divers masters were hardened rather to suffer their servants to perish for want of fitt meanes and applications then by seeking reliefe to fall into the hands of griping and avaricious men.

It was decided that the physician could be arrested and hailed into court if he was accused of excessive charges, the act of 1646 specifying the county court.[11] Although, in 1660, a sop was thrown to the profession when the law permitted " Physitians and Chyrurgions " to collect against a dead man's estate, the physician and his fees were of constant interest to the assembly, and the law of 1639 was continually reenacted. Evidently physicians and chirurgeons did not cut their rates sufficiently; for the Assembly passed a law in 1736 setting the fees for services.[12]

[11] Hening, *Virginia*, I, pp. 316-317.
[12] *Ibid.*, II, p. 26.

MEDICAL REGULATIONS AND SOCIETIES

The Massachusetts act of 1649 was more comprehensive and reflected public suspicion of the profession.

Foreasmuch as the Law of God allows no man to impair the life or limbs, of any person, but in a judicial way. It is therefore Ordered, That no person or persons whatsoever imployed at any times, about the bodyes of men, women or children for preservation of life or health, as Chirurgeons, Midwives, Physicians or others, presume to exercise or put forth, any act, contrary to the known approved rules of art, in each mistery or occupation, nor exercise any force, violence, or cruelty upon, or towards, the body of any, whether young or old (no not in the most difficult and desperate cases) without the advice and consent of such as are skilful in the same art (if such may be had) or at least of some of the wisest and gravest then present and consent of the patient or patients if they be mente compotes, much less contrary to such advice and consent upon such severe punishment, as the nature of the case may deserve, which Law nevertheless, is not intended to discourage any from all use of their skill, but rather incourage & direct them.[13]

This Massachusetts law, reenacted in 1660, was the basis, almost word for word, for the New York law of 1664.[14]

The first law to make provision for examining prospective practitioners was "*An Act to regulate the Practice of Physick and Surgery in the City of New York*" passed in 1760. The introduction stated that many ignorant and unskilled persons preyed upon the sick of the city. To stop this, all who wished to practice were to be examined by one of the Council, the Judge of the Supreme Court, the King's Attorney General and the Mayor or any three of them. These in turn were to call in examiners whom they regarded as competent. Without the "Testimonial" of a successful

---

[13] *Massachusetts, The Colonial Laws of* . . . , pp. 137-138.
[14] *New York, The Colonial Laws of* . . . *from 1664 to the Revolution* . . . (4 volumes, Albany, 1894), I, p. 27.

examination, practitioners were to be fined £50 for each offence, one-half to go to the informer and one-half to the poor. As usual, this law exempted those already in practice.[15]

The statute affecting New York City served as a model for the more comprehensive law passed by New Jersey in 1772. Two judges of the Supreme Court with the aid of physicians were required to examine the applicant. A fine of five pounds was assessed for practicing without a license. This penalty did not apply, however, to those who performed services gratuitously or to skilful persons called into the state for special reasons. In addition, the law required that all medical bills be written in English and be subject to taxation. The medicine-show men were hard hit by a £20 fine on all " Mountebanks " on the stage who sold medicine.[16]

More stringent regulations were contained in the laws passed shortly under the Republic. Their administration was generally placed in the hands of medical societies or boards of examiners established by various methods of appointment. In nearly all cases a diploma of a recognized college was accepted as sufficient qualification. The first medical society, with the right to regulate medical practice, was the Massachusetts Medical Society. In 1781 Samuel Danforth, John French, Edward A. Holyoke, the Isaac Rands, Senior and Junior, Cotton Tuffs and John Warren, and others were incorporated with powers to regulate practice.[17] The law detailed the various offices, duties of the officers, the society's right to sue and be sued and kindred

[15] *Ibid.*, IV, pp. 455-456.

[16] *New Jersey, Acts of . . . 1702-1776*, Compiled by Samuel Allenson (Burlington, 1776), pp. 376-377; *New Jersey Acts of . . . 1800*. Rev. Ed. William Patterson (Newark, 1800), p. 79. This law, which expired in 1777, was reënacted in 1783 and 1786.

[17] Massachusetts Medical Society, *Medical Papers*, 1790, Pref. pp. viii-ix.

legal niceties. The President and Fellows were authorized to examine all candidates for the license. If the President and Fellows refused to serve, they were subject to a £100 fine.[18] When Harvard College opened its medical department the following year, it was decided that, since the requirements were satisfactory, Harvard graduates should be admitted to practice without examination.[19]

One of the distinguishing features of the Massachusetts Medical Society was its list of recommended readings for the prospective candidates, this list being required of the society by the law of 1789. The statute also required the applicant to pay *reasonable* fees. The President was protected against the £100 fine for failure or refusal to examine by providing that the candidate sue the censors (board of examiners) who refused him examination.[20] Finally in 1803 the law was codified and continued in force for some time. Five censors were to be appointed to examine the candidates, who should be admitted to practice three months after the vote of the society; as the state grew, new districts could be marked off; and, the fellows were exempted from military duty.[21]

By laws of 1818 and 1819 a degree from any college admitted a physician to practice, but if he wished to collect debts, he had to be a Harvard graduate or hold a license from the Massachusetts Medical Society.[22] According to the by-laws of the society for 1832, the candidate had to give evidence that he had studied three years with an approved doctor; possessed a knowledge of Latin, geometry and ex-

[18] *Massachusetts, The Laws of* ... *1780-1807* (3 volumes, Boston, 1808), III, pp. 140-143.
[19] Massachusetts Medical Society, *Medical Papers*, II, p. 25.
[20] *Massachusetts, Laws of* ... *1780-1807*, III, pp. 144-145.
[21] *Ibid.*, pp. 145-146.
[22] *Massachusetts, Laws of* ... *1818* (Boston, 1818), p. 540; *ibid., 1819* (Boston, 1819), pp. 179-180.

perimental philosophy; and had completed certain prescribed reading. He had to submit to an examination on all phases of medicine and be approved by a majority vote.[23] These laws were rendered innocuous some years later by the repeal of the clause of 1818 which prevented debt-collection by non-licensed practitioners. When Maine was separated from Massachusetts in 1821, its medical society received a charter similar to Massachusetts, with the substitution of Bowdoin College for Harvard Medical School as the state medical college and the requirement that all doctors belong to the society.[24]

Although the Connecticut Medical Society (1792) had these rights to regulate the practice of medicine, in 1797 it varied the procedure of examination by having the state committee examine candidates recommended by county committees. The fee was the usual ten dollars, returnable if the candidate failed.[25] Yale College established its medical department under the direction of the state medical society. By the codified law of 1821, the state required professors and four members of its medical society to comprise a board of examiners of candidates. It also provided that unlicensed physicians who had begun practice since 1800 could not collect debts.[26] One year later the state interceded to help the society collect back dues by providing that suits would be begun against delinquent members in six months.[27] With

[23] *Massachusetts Medical Society, Acts of Incorporation and Acts Regulating the Practice of Physic and Surgery with the By-Laws and Orders of the* . . . (Boston, 1832), pp. 404-5.

[24] *Medical Society of Maine, Incorporation, Constitution, By-Laws &c., of the* . . . (Bath, 1824), pp. 1-7; *Maine, Acts of* . . . *1821-1834* (2 volumes, Portland, 1834), II, pp. 1272-1273.

[25] Connecticut Medical Society, *Transactions, 1792-1829*, Pref. vi-ix, p. 49.

[26] *Connecticut, Laws of* . . . Rev. Ed. 1821 (Hartford, 1821), pp. 322-323.

[27] *Connecticut, Laws of* . . . *1822* (Hartford, 1824), pp. 22-23.

little additional legislation Connecticut continued its medical control until it, too, repealed the provision that only licensed practitioners could collect debts.[28]

The various acts, passed to regulate the practice of medicine in New York State, illustrate the growth and decline of such legislation. For some time after the law to regulate practice in New York City, the state went uncontrolled. In 1792 a law providing a fine of seven pounds and non-collection of debts for unlicensed practitioners, but permitting practice to recipients of college degrees, was enacted for New York City and County.[29] In 1797 and 1801 laws were passed continuing the chancellor and judges, assisted by physicians, as examiners, and outlawing unlicensed practitioners unless they had practiced since 1795 or unless they held college degrees.[30] What actually happened under this statute appears in *An Act to enable William Firley to practice physic and surgery* because a number of " respectable inhabitants " of towns in Suffolk County petitioned it.[31]

Finally in 1806 the legislature decided to place medical regulation in the hands of a state society. County societies were organized and their delegates were to meet once a year as the state society. The county societies had charge of admission to the profession, but if a candidate felt that he had been treated unfairly, he could appeal to the state body. The usual requirements were noted for candidates. Then the law outlawed practitioners without licenses who had begun practice *after* January 1805.[32] After many changes,

[28] *Connecticut Laws of . . . 1836-1837* (Hartford, 1837), p. 109. Omitted from 1834.
[29] *New York, Laws of . . . 1775-1792* (2 volumes, N. Y., 1792), II, pp. 425-426.
[30] *New York, Laws of . . . 1777-1801* (2 volumes, Albany, 1802), I, pp. 449-452.
[31] *New York, Laws of . . . 1804* (Albany, 1804), pp. 407-408.
[32] *New York, Laws of . . . 1806*, pp. 437-444.

the law in 1813 was again codified; and at the same time it was weakened by a clause permitting practice with herbs of American growth.[33] By a general revision of the medical code in 1827, practically all provisions of the old laws were reenacted. With the exception of a clause refusing to recognize courses taken at the Rutgers Medical College (the school founded in opposition to the College of Physicians and Surgeons of New York City), no important changes were made.[34]

About 1835 a wave of repeal of state medical laws began. The skepticism concerning the efficacy of legal control resulted from the attacks of irregular doctors upon regular practices, and the failure of the profession, working under a monopoly, to justify by its works its favored position. After many efforts repeal of the regulatory function of the New York State Medical Society was carried in 1844. As in other states, this did not mean abolition of the state medical society, but merely the repeal of the penalty clauses of the medical laws. After repeal, quacks could be prosecuted only on charges of either malpractice or gross ignorance.[35] In the course of the debate on medical laws one Senator said, " The people of this state have been bled long enough in their bodies and pockets, and it was [sic] time they should do as the men of the Revolution did: resolve to set down [sic] and enjoy the freedom for which they bled." [36] The Medical Society of the State of New York accepted the changes philosophically. Its special committee approved the action of the legislature because the regulations had never been fully

[33] *New York, Laws of* . . . Rev. Ed. (2 volumes, Albany, 1813), II, pp. 219 *et seq.*

[34] *New York, Laws of* . . . *1827*, Rev. Ed. (Albany, 1827), pp. 298 *et seq.*

[35] *New York, Laws of* . . . *1844*, pp. 406-407.

[36] *New York Medical Society, Proceedings, 1844-1846* (Albany, 1846), App., p. 71, 1845, quoted from the *Albany Evening Atlas*.

enforced and because the committee believed that progress in medical science did not depend upon laws.[37]

The societies of the District of Columbia and Illinois respectively illustrate both the development of a society with legal control of practice and the vicissitudes of early organization. In 1813 the physicians of the city of Washington met in a memorial service for Benjamin Rush. Four years later in September 1817, a meeting was announced in the *National Intelligencer* to fight "pretenders."[38] At the end of two years, the society received its charter, including the right to regulate the practice of medicine, from Congress. In 1836, however, this right was invalidated by the Supreme Court.[39] In most parts of the country if the courts did not intervene to defend irregular practitioners, faulty legislation enabled the quack to escape punishment. Although it is by no means typical, the history of the Medical Society of Illinois is amusing. It was chartered in 1819. The legislature decided to void the charter in 1821, but four years later the society was revived. Finally in 1826, the legislature changed its mind for the last time and abandoned the attempt to control medical practice through a state society.[40]

After using medical societies to regulate medical practices, the states turned to medical boards, variously appointed.

[37] *Ibid.*, pp. 54-57. An examination particularly of the Albany Society, an active body, shows that constant efforts brought few results.

The following is a list of the states which established medical societies with the right to regulate: New Hampshire, 1791; Maryland, 1799; New Jersey, laws of 1816 and 1830; South Carolina, society founded in 1792 but right to regulate granted in 1817; Delaware, 1819; Vermont, 1820; District of Columbia, 1819; Mississippi, 1829; Indiana, 1825.

[38] *Medical Society of the District of Columbia, 1817-1909*, pp. 1-3.

[39] *Ibid.*, pp. 10-11 quoting Cranch's *Reports*, V, pp. 62-71.

[40] *Illinois, Laws of . . . 1820-1821* (Vandalia, 1821), pp. 3-4; *ibid., 1824-1825* (Vandalia, 1825), pp. 111-113; *Ibid., 1826* (Vandalia, 1826), p. 75.

Ohio combined the two methods of control. Following laws in 1811 and 1817, in 1820 the legislature granted physicians the right to organize district societies whenever ten or more physicians asked permission, rate agreements being banned. These societies set up boards, subject to the state officials, to pass upon applicants for licenses to practice. The fines affecting unlicensed practitioners, however, were repealed and Ohio's " medical convention " was powerless to stop the activities of quack doctors.[41]

The normal procedure in creating boards of medical examiners was for the legislature or the governor to appoint a group of men for a district. The number of examiners in each district varied from three to seven, with a majority vote deciding. By an act of 1820, Louisiana named five physicians and one apothecary for the Eastern District of the state. This board was to examine all candidates for a license, but it was required to accept the diploma of any medical college in the United States. The president of the board was further required to supply the attorney general with a list of unlicensed practitioners for prosecution.[42] Subsequently in 1840, the medical board received permission to fine unlicensed practitioners.[43] Alabama, in 1823, likewise set up boards of examiners with similar rights and restrictions.[44] At a later date, it permitted Thomsonians to practice on the condition that they use no allopathic medicines.[45]

[41] *Ohio, Acts of ... 1810-1811* (Zanesville, 1811), pp. 19-23; *ibid., 1816-1817* (Columbus, 1817), pp. 195-201; *ibid., 1819-1820* (Columbus, 1820), p. 162.

[42] *Louisiana, Acts of . . . 1820*, pp. 30-32.

[43] *Louisiana, Acts of . . . 1845* (New Orleans, 1845), p. 68.

[44] *Alabama, Acts of . . . 1823* (Cahawba, 1823), pp. 45-47; *ibid., 1827* (Tuscaloosa, 1827), pp. 77-78.

[45] *Alabama, Digest of the Laws of . . . John G. Aiken* (Phila., 1833), p. 340.

MEDICAL REGULATIONS AND SOCIETIES   213

Besides Florida [46] and Texas,[47] Georgia was the only other state to rely upon medical boards. Its law of 1825, evidently fell into disuse, for it was revived in 1839 in an amusing bit of legislation, which forbade the board to act against Thomsonians or "any other practitioners of medicine in this State." [48] In 1847, the state went further than any other in protecting quacks when it set up the "Botanic Medical Board of Physicians" with the provision that only graduates of the botanic school could collect fees from botanic practices.[49] Virginia, by an act of 1813, provided a forty-dollar fine for all those practicing without a license.[50]

Regulation of medical practice, by medical societies or by medical boards, was ineffective. At the beginning of the Republic the high standards of the medical societies were difficult to maintain because of the poor work in the medical schools. Most of the laws set dates permitting practitioners of that date to continue in practice. The upshot was that the immediate passage of a law worked no hardship, but as time passed and certain people were prosecuted and even barred from practice, public opinion forced a change to a later date. Frequently, it was possible to appeal from regulating bodies to the state legislature, and such an appeal was successful in the case of William Firley in New York State. The *Oglethorpe Medical* and *Surgical Journal* said that in Georgia any one could appeal to the legislature from the

---

[46] *Florida Territory, Acts of the Legislative Council of . . . 1824* (Tallahassee, 1825), pp. 277-278. *Ibid., 1828* (Tallahassee, 1828), pp. 258-260; and Duval, John P., *Compilation of 1839* (Tallahassee, 1839), p. 368.

[47] *Texas, Laws of . . . General and Private,* 1848 (2 volumes, 1848, p. p.), II, p. 21.

[48] *Georgia, Acts of . . . 1830* (Milledgeville, 1831), pp. 245; *ibid., 1839* (Milledgeville, 1840), pp. 187-188.

[49] *Ibid., 1847* (Milledgeville, 1848), pp. 234-237.

[50] *Virginia, Acts of . . . 1813* (Richmond, 1813), p. 10.

Board of Examiners and get a license.[51] The passage of laws restricting medical practice reached its highest point in 1825; and thereafter, due to the attacks of the empirics and the realization by the profession of the futility of regulations, practically all laws were repealed.

Besides repeal in Connecticut, Massachusetts and New York, Maine emasculated its law by permitting collection of medical debts on presentation of a certificate of good character from a selectman.[52] In 1843, the Monroe County Medical Society of New York submitted a report to the state medical society favoring repeal of existing fines. This report stated that Maryland, South Carolina, Delaware and Indiana had repealed the enforcing provisions of their laws.[53] The *Boston Medical and Surgical Journal* summed up the situation in the same year as follows: eight states never had any regulatory laws; ten states had abolished their laws; four still had laws; and four states had not replied. Of the four which did not reply, namely Arkansas, Illinois, Michigan and Delaware, Michigan alone had a law providing prosecution for malpractice of " persons holding themselves out to the public as physicians." [54] According to an investigation by the American Medical Association in 1849, only New Jersey and the District of Columbia had laws regulating the practice of medicine.[55]

HEALTH REGULATIONS

In addition to regulating the practice of medicine, the legislatures tried to protect public health. Even in colonial times and later under the republic laws were passed setting

---

[51] *Oglethorpe Medical and Surgical Journal* (Savannah, 1858-1859), I, pp. 84-85; *Alabama, Laws of . . . 1849-1850* (Tuscaloosa, 1850), p. 531. The state legislature allowed ten men to practice without a license.

[52] *Maine, Public Acts of . . . 1838* (Augusta, 1838), p. 510.

[53] *New York Medical Society, Proceedings, 1844-1846*, App., pp. 37-46.

[54] *Boston Medical and Surgical Journal*, XXVIII, 1843, p. 323.

[55] *American Medical Association, Transactions*, 1849, pp. 326 *et seq.*

up boards of health and health offices, staffed by doctors, in order to inspect ships in seaport towns or to regulate intercourse with infected areas and keep down "nuisances" or disease-provoking conditions within the cities. These health officers were selected by three different means; the governor of the state was empowered to select them; the mayor and city council could be constituted a board of health to select the proper officials; or the townspeople could select the health board in their selection. Of the three methods the first was the most common and the last was unusual. These health officers generally had the power to stop vessels at quarantine, to inspect them, to require the disinfection of the vessels, to burn filth or infected clothing, to collect fees from the passengers and crew, and lastly, after finding matters satisfactory, to give the ship master a bill of health which permitted him to advance to the city. In the case of towns, the health officers had the right to force the removal of dirt, regulate the cleaning of privies and to establish pesthouses to care for those ill with infectious diseases. The health officers, in conjunction with the inspectors, city council or governor as the case might be, could declare a given district under quarantine and prevent intercourse with it and lay down penalties for the violation of the laws. They received their pay either in percentages of fees or cash from receipts from the vessels which they inspected or in salaries from the state. Generally the health offices of maritime cities and towns were self-supporting. In these towns control was extended to seamen and lodging houses whose owners were required, under various penalties for nonconformance, to report all infected sailors. The sailors were confined to the pesthouses or lazarettoes which were constructed for their care.[56]

[56] *Pennsylvania, Laws of the Commonwealth of* . . . *1700-1801*, Ed. A. J. Dallas (4 volumes, Phila., 1795-1801), III, pp. 553-573. This law, passed in 1794 is a good example. All states had these laws, and the summary is based upon an examination of them.

Besides the general laws dealing with health offices, regulations were passed to protect the community against smallpox. We have already explained that inoculation is the introduction of the variolous matter whereas vaccination is the introduction of cowpox. Before Jenner's discovery, inoculation had been regulated. Georgia, for example, provided in an act of 1768 that all persons carelessly introducing variolus would be fined, but granted to magistrates jurisdiction over inoculation. It further provided that hospitals for inoculation should be eight hundred yards from the road and that infected houses should be advertised by signs.[57]

When people had to rely upon inoculation, there was always the danger of an epidemic. Vaccination removed this danger and made possible the removal of the disease. Obviously, it took some time to wear down popular antipathy and fear, but by 1830 vaccination was not only generally permitted but widely fostered by the state governments. First in the effort to make vaccination universal, Massachusetts provided in 1810 that:

it shall be the duty of every town district, and plantation within this commonwealth, wherein no board of health shall be established by law, . . . to choose, . . . three or more suitable persons, whose duty it shall be to superintend the inoculation of inhabitants of such town, district or plantation, with the cowpox.[58]

Between this time and 1850, New Hampshire required vaccination in 1835,[59] while Rhode Island, Virginia, Maine, Georgia and Louisiana provided free vaccination. Two states, New York and New Jersey, incorporated Vaccine Institutes in New York City and Paterson respectively, which offered free vaccination and were excellent examples of the

[57] *Georgia, Colonial Records of* . . . XIX, pt. 1, pp. 22-28.

[58] *Massachusetts, Laws of* . . . *1810* (n. p., n. d.), p. 204. It contained the provision that the towns were to pay.

[59] *New Hampshire, Laws of* . . . *1835* (Concord, 1835), pp. 182-183.

work carried on elsewhere by philanthropic citizens.⁶⁰ It might be said that within thirty years of the introduction of Jenner's discovery the United States had freed itself from the constant menace of smallpox. In this achievement the medical profession had taken the initiative, but success had been assured by the cooperation of state legislatures.

Occasionally, the legislatures were faced with situations as grave if not graver than yellow fever and smallpox. In 1832 Asiatic Cholera reached America, after giving advance notice by sweeping through Europe. We have seen how the doctors published precautions and how the weekly magazinies were called into being to mitigate the epidemic. In such circumstances, it became necessary to pass strict laws providing for effective quarantine and general regulations. In 1832, New York enacted a comprehensive law. It provided: (1) quarantine for vessels from afflicted regions and for those districts where the disease had spread rapidly within the state; (2) health boards in the cities and towns with power to establish quarantine, make regulations for health, raise money and issue warrants to enforce their rules; (3) payment of expenses by counties and states, according to agency in curing them; and (4) continuation of this law until 1833 unless the Governor ended it by proclamation.⁶¹ Besides New York, Rhode Island practically proclaimed martial law when it gave the governor the right to use ships to inspect for Asiatic Cholera, to provide hospitals and to enforce regulations, and to take "requisite" money from the treasury for such purposes.⁶² In this fashion the nation prepared for one of its worst epidemics.

⁶⁰ *New York, Laws of* . . . *1844*, pp. 101-102; *New Jersey, Laws of* . . . *1831-1832* (Trenton, 1832), pp. 34-35.

⁶¹ *New York, Laws of* . . . *1832* (Albany, 1832), pp. 581-584; *ibid.*, *1835*, p. 90; *ibid.*, *1833* (Albany, 1833), p. 305.

⁶² *Rhode Island, Public Laws of* . . . *1831-1833* (Providence, 1833), pp. 804-805.

THE ORGANIZATION OF MEDICAL SOCIETIES

After this examination of laws passed to regulate the practice of medicine and laws designed to improve the public health, we may now consider the various activities of the medical societies. Although such societies had existed in colonial times, it is clear that the desire of the states to establish agencies to enforce medical legislation was an impetus to their development. By the time the state deprived them of their regulatory powers, they were firmly entrenched in professional life. They, therefore, continued to play an important part in promoting professional spirit; in fact, it was after the repeal of the regulatory clauses that the societies found an outlet in a national organization. It is now possible to examine them with regard to their organization and their efforts to enforce ethics without legal power, to sum up their difficulties, and finally, to give the history of the American Medical Association in its early years.

The medical societies may be divided into three groups: first, those which were granted regulatory functions by the states; second, those which were voluntary organizations without such powers; and third, those which were interested in scientific or in specialized phases of medicine. The first two groups had similar organizations. The purely scientific were confined to the large cities; the specialized groups were interested in only one phase of medicine. Once a year, delegates from counties or districts—New York and Connecticut had counties as the lesser unit whereas Massachusetts, New Jersey and Ohio had districts—gathered at the state capital to carry out their work. County or district societies met as frequently as they desired, which might be once or twice a year or even bi-monthly, depending upon the activity of the group.[63] The specialized societies, with the exception of

---

[63] *Vermont, Acts of . . . 1829* (Middlebury, 1831), p. 71. The Medical Society of Caledonia County was authorized to hold its semi-annual

such organizations as the Society of Superintendents of the Insane, met more frequently than state societies, monthly meetings being usual. The dues of state societies seldom exceeded two dollars per year. According to the New York law of 1806 the dues could not exceed three dollars; those of the Maryland Medical and Chirurgical Faculty were five dollars; in 1800, Connecticut raised its duties from two to four dollars.[64] Some of the New York county societies also charged an initiation fee. The Albany county society charged three dollars, whereas the Mohawk and Buffalo Village Societies charged one dollar, if a dissertation were given, and two dollars without it.[65] The College of Physicians of Philadelphia, because it was a select group, had a £10 initiation fee. These fees and the examination charges were usually assigned by law to the libraries of the societies.

As a rule when the delegates from these local societies attended the meeting of the state society, they paid their own expenses.[66] At the opening or closing of the state meeting, depending upon the desire of the individual society, the president or the person appointed by the previous meeting

meetings at such places as a majority of the members present should direct.

[64] *New York, Laws of . . . 1806* (Albany, 1906), pp. 437-444; *Maryland, Laws of . . .* Kilty, Harris and Watkins, V, Sess. 1816, ch. 169; *Connecticut Medical Society, Transactions of the . . . 1792-1829* (Hartford, 1884), Pref., pp. vi-ix.

[65] Willard, Sylvester D., *Annals of the Medical Society of the County of Albany, 1806-1851* (Albany, 1851), p. 5; Kellert, Ellis, *Early Medical History of the Mohawk Valley* (Schenectady, 1932), p. 21; Medical Society of the Village of Buffalo, The Constitution and Bye-Laws of the . . . Adopted July 16, 1831. Ms. in Buffalo Historical Society.

[66] County of Greene, Records of the Bye-Laws and Proceedings of the Medical Society of the . . . State of New York, April 4, 1808–May 30, 1837. Ms. in New York Academy of Medicine, p. 7; John Ely was allowed five dollars expenses; *Otsego Medical Society, Bye-Laws of the . . . 1820* (Cooperstown, N. Y., 1821, p. 3; ten dollars expenses were allowed.

gave an address. These speeches were seldom interesting. Favorite topics were education, quackery and recent improvements in medicine. Occasionally an address of unusual merit startled the profession. Such was the speech of Jacob Bigelow entitled " Discourse on Self-Limited Diseases ", delivered to the Massachusetts Medical Society in 1835, of which Oliver Wendell Holmes said; " This remarkable essay had more influence on medical practice in America than any other similar brief treatise." [67] Bigelow pointed out that the profession in the early years of the nineteenth century had made progress in diagnosis of disease. He called attention, however, to the lack of progress in therapeutics. The profession, he insisted, had introduced few new remedies, cures being effected largely because certain diseases are self-limited. He wished the profession to turn its attention to these diseases, seemingly beyond human remedy, to classify and to experiment with new methods of attack.[68] After lectures, such as this one, the medical societies settled down to discussions or reports or to their special duties. The most important function of a society was the regulation of the practice of medicine. Since many states did not grant this function to the societies or had repealed the original grant, as time went on the societies turned to an intensive examination of the status of the medical profession.

ENFORCEMENT OF MEDICAL ETHICS

Whether or not the state regulated the practice of medicine, the societies attempted to establish standards of conduct

[67] Burrage, Walter L., *A History of the Massachusetts Medical Society . . . 1781-1922* (Boston, 1923), p. 1.

[68] Bigelow, Jacob, *Discourse on Self-Limited Diseases* (Boston, 1835), pp. 7-8. This difficulty of arriving at a more positive (or scientific) cure of disease is recognized by modern scientists. The self-limitation of disease plays a prominent part in Sinclair Lewis's novel, *Arrowsmith*, in which the statistical results of his serum are examined by Dr. Raymond Pearl, who is an eminent professor at Johns Hopkins University.

for their members and to hold the members to them. Although Percival's *Code of Ethics* was the criterion of professional behavior, the by-laws of all societies served a similar purpose. Less elaborate, they briefly covered the conduct of the "respectable" practitioner. In their efforts to enforce the state laws and ethical codes, the societies spent considerable fruitless effort. It is obvious that enforcement of state or medical rules depended upon the character of the members of the societies. Briefly, Connecticut and Massachusetts were the most active state groups; in New York State, where enforcement was by county societies, the Medical Society of Albany County had a similar record.

The common methods of controlling the personal conduct of physicians were: first, refusal to admit to the profession; second, expulsion for immoral conduct; third, expulsion for the sale of secret " nostrums " of any sort; fourth, expulsion for association with quacks or irregulars; fifth, expulsion for violation of laws; and, sixth, a miscellany of controls by means of investigation and publication of facts. Unfortunately the societies did not keep records of candidates who failed the qualifying examination. There is no reason, when one considers the numbers admitted to the profession, to believe that the examinations were difficult. On the contrary admission to young men of good moral character, twenty-one years of age, with the minimum educational requirements was easy. Occasionally a candidate was refused on moral grounds. In 1836 Joel Devine was refused a diploma by the Dutchess County Medical Society. As a result, a quarrel within the profession ensued, and the society did not meet from 1845 to 1854. Since the court intervened to secure Devine a diploma, the effort was unsuccessful.[69] On

[69] Bayley, G. C., *An Historical Address delivered before the Dutchess County Medical Society at its Centennial Meeting, January 10, 1906* (Poughkeepsie, N. Y., 1906), pp. 6-7.

the grounds that he advertised, the Albany society refused Dr. V. B. Lockrow membership.[70] Despite a few other cases, this means of controlling the profession was unimportant.

Expulsion was used. At this time, several states made abortion a criminal offense. At least one society considered it a violation of medical ethics. The Medical Society of Oneida County expelled N. W. Smith for performing an abortion. Although the Court did not find it an indictable offense, it upheld the medical society; the fact that Smith was also guilty of adultery may have added weight to the case against him. Similarly, Andrew Winer was removed from the Greene County (New York) Society for "high crimes and misdemeanors" in 1810 without explanation of the broad phraseology.[71]

The manufacture and sale of secret medicines was the most common charge against physicians. Doctors caught between poverty and a discovery of some value often succumbed to the temptation to patent their prescriptions. The by-laws of all societies required giving such information to the profession. The best-known case is that of Elisha Perkins of Connecticut, who was expelled in 1797 because he patented "painted metallic instruments pretending that they possess inherent powers of curing many diseases, and that they were an invention of his own." He did not recant and as late as 1836 the sale was being carried on.[72]

Massachusetts expelled Dr. Lyman B. Sarbin of Wrentham for his *Peges Vegetable Cyrup* and *Dr. Lee's Gravel Specific*.[73] Albany expelled Dr. Elias Willard for refusal to

[70] Willard, *op. cit.*, p. 145.

[71] *New York Medical Society, Proceedings of . . . 1834-1835* (Albany, 1835), pp. 379-388; Medical Society of Greene County, Minutes, p. 10.

[72] Connecticut Medical Society, *Transactions*, 1796, p. 40; 1797, p. 50. *Boston Medical and Surgical Journal*, XV, 1836, p. 162. *Cf. supra*, p. 200.

[73] Massachusetts Medical Society, *Medical Papers*, VII, pp. 88-90.

reveal his cure for cancer and scrofula.[74] Usually the erring member could regain his rights by disclosing the nature of his preparation. In 1800, the following appeared in the *Transactions* of the Connecticut Medical Society: "Personally appeared before me the subscriber, a Justice of Peace of Hartford County, Mr. Mark Newell, Physician, and made oath that the articles above enumerated are those and the only articles made use of in his Jaundice Pills or family Physic." It was signed by Daniel Rockwell, the Justice of Peace.[75] Reports, such as those made to the New York County Medical Society, as well as articles which appeared in the medical journals constitute a record of patent medicines.

Removal of a member for consorting with quacks was not so frequent as for selling secret medicines. Benjamin Waterhouse, who was credited with the introduction of vaccination into America, was charged with excessive sympathy for herbalists. His name and fame prevented drastic action by the Massachusetts society; and, although he espoused the cause of Thomson and his lobelia leaf, his name was carried on the society rolls from the day of his resignation in 1806 until 1832.[76]

No case brings out the confusion of issues so well as that of Dr. J. S. Bartlett of the Massachusetts Medical Society. Briefly, Bartlett, a member of the society, was associated with two non-members, Dr. Patrick Kearney and a Dr. Williams, famous for his cures or reported cures of the blind. Bartlett, contesting his removal from the society, offered as justification that Dr. Kearney was a regular physician whose Catholicism had prevented the society from asking him to join. In addition Bartlett claimed that Williams *did* cure the blind and that he, Bartlett, was within his oath

[74] Willard, *op. cit.*, p. 24.
[75] Connecticut Medical Society, *Transactions*, 1800, p. 78.
[76] Burrage, *op. cit.*, p. 89.

to support the laws " so far as they are consistent with morality and the general good of mankind." He embarrassed the society by mentioning the support which Dr. John C. Warren had given Graham's dietary reforms, not exactly a parallel case, among other indiscretions of his judges. He exposed the fact that the Massachusetts General Hospital used Swaim's Panacea, a highly advertised patent medicine. After expulsion, Bartlett petitioned the state legislature to revoke the charter of the medical society.[77] His death, in 1840, ended the dispute. His contentions, however, disclosed the dubious practices of many of the Boston profession.

The by-laws required every member to report his delinquent fellows. When this method of control broke down, committees, such as one in New York City in 1830, might be appointed to investigate the conduct of the members. One of the common misdemeanors which it found was the practice of soliciting business in venereal cases.[78] New Hampshire expelled a member for writing an article in the *Congregational Journal*,[79] publication being limited to medical journals. Control of quacks was attempted by impeaching committees, personal warnings to unlicensed practitioners and the publication of lists of qualified physicians in newspapers, but none of these proved effective.[80]

In addition to these efforts, the minutes of societies contain constant references to petitions to the state legislatures for medical laws or revision of existing laws. To further

[77] *Boston Medical and Surgical Journal*, XIV, pp. 240-243, 256-258, 277-292, 282-303; XX, p. 243.

[78] *Medical Society of New York County, Minutes of . . . 1807-1831* (New York, 1831), p. 427 and pp. 430-431. Although venereal diseases are not mentioned as such, the wording makes them obvious.

[79] *New Hampshire Medical Society, Records of the . . . from its organization in 1791 to the year 1854* (Concord, 1911), pp. 341-342, 350.

[80] Willard, *op. cit.*, pp. 72 and 142; Medical Society of Connecticut, *Transactions*, 1799, p. 72.

MEDICAL REGULATIONS AND SOCIETIES 225

its ends, the profession, in several cases, resorted to an economic threat. The clergy, who were recipients of free medical attention, occasionally seem to have turned a penny by endorsing quack medicines. At least three state medical societies resolved to discontinue free attention unless clergymen withdrew their endorsement of patent medicines. The Connecticut Medical Society did not mince words when it said,

Whereas it is believed to be the custom of the regular physicians of the State, at the present time, to render *medical services* to clergymen and their families gratuitously,

And whereas it is believed that as a class of citizens (their education, intelligence, and standing considered), they do more than any other class in the community to embarrass the legitimate influence of the medical profession;

Therefore, Resolved, That as a rule we adopt the practice of charging clergymen the same fees as other citizens, except in cases of misfortune or inability, which would render it burdensome to make a just compensation for services rendered.[81]

OTHER ACTIVITIES OF THE SOCIETIES

Next to combating the quacks and supervising the activities of their own members, the medical societies were most interested in the educational system. Occasionally a medical society petitioned the state legislature to charter a college in its district. In 1822 the Berkshire Medical Association petitioned the Massachusetts legislature for such a college and a grant of money to build it. The college opened its doors in 1824.[82] After the legislature granted permission to the Connecticut Medical Society to establish a medical college, the

---

[81] *Ibid.*, 1848, p. 5. Other societies were the Medical Association of South Carolina, *Minutes, 1850*, p. 20; and Indiana Medical Convention, *Minutes, 1849*, p. 10.

[82] Berkshire Medical Association, Minutes, Ms. in the Berkshire Athenâeum, p. 5.

school was organized in 1811 in connection with Yale College but subject to the society.[83] An examining committee of the medical society attended examinations and passed upon the qualifications of the candidates. This was the only successful case of such a union.[24] The demands for salaried professors, longer terms, more careful preparation and curricular changes occupied much of the societies' time. The effect of these speeches and committee reports may have been slight; nevertheless, when members of the faculties could get together for three hours' discussion of educational problems, as they did in 1848 at the meeting of the national association, a valuable interchange of ideas inevitably took place.[85]

In order to keep up with new ideas, the medical societies collected libraries. State legislatures usually allocated yearly dues, after the ordinary expenses had been paid, to this end. The Massachusetts Medical Society began collecting a library as early as 1787.[86] The Medical Society of South Carolina in 1850 had a collection of 2398 volumes.[87] In 1853 the Worcester District Medical Society of Massachusetts reported 450 volumes.[88] Very few other libraries attained this size, and probably the majority were nearer the seventy-six volumes of the Albany County society in 1831.[89] Since few

[83] Connecticut Medical Society, *Transactions*, 1810, p. 161.

[84] *Ibid.*, p. 7. In 1848 the committee noted improvement in the literary and professional equipment of candidates. In South Carolina such a college was proposed, but the society lost much of its power and split into factions, the latter as a result of the school.

[85] Warren, Edward, *Life of John Collins Warren* (2 volumes, Boston, 1860), II, p. 15.

[86] Massachusetts Medical Society, *Medical Papers*, 1790, Pref. iv-v.

[87] South Carolina Medical Association, *Minutes and Proceedings, 1849-1850* (Charleston), p. 61.

[88] *Worcester District Medical Society, By-Laws of the . . . with a list of members and catalogue of library* (Worcester [1853?]), pp. 22-23.

[89] Willard, *op. cit.*, p. 103.

societies kept records or printed information regarding the libraries, we may assume that they were small;[90] some may have been like that of the Medical Society of the District of Columbia in which Toner, in 1866, found but one volume. The other gifts had gone the way of most collections when their safekeeping is not insured.[91] In addition to reference books, the chief interest was in periodicals, thus in 1824 the Medical Society of New York City had the *American Medical Repository, New York Medical and Physical Journal, New England Medical and Surgical Journal, New York Monthly Magazine, Philadelphia Medical and Physical Journal,* and eight foreign journals on its list of recommended purchases.[92]

The Medical and Chirurgical Faculty of Maryland had laws governing its library. Prior to 1854 the library was open from five until seven from May to September and from three-thirty to five-thirty during the rest of the year. After 1854 it was open from ten in the morning until ten at night. Careful laws, such as fines, regulated borrowing, and no books were issued until fines were paid; no loans were permitted to outsiders; and a requirement was made of endorsement by two directors of the society in order to borrow rare books.[93] The necessity for well-drawn rules indicates a library of good size, catering to an interested group.

An occasional activity of the medical societies was to award a prize for the best essay on some medical topic. The Boylston Medical Society in Boston gave a first prize of twenty-

[90] *Cf. supra,* Chapter III, pp. 73-74.

[91] *Medical Society of the District of Columbia, 1817-1909,* pp. 40-42.

[92] *Medical Society of New York County, Minutes, 1807-1831,* 1824, pp. 291-292.

[93] *Medical and Chirurgical Faculty of Maryland, Act of Incorporation of* . . . (Baltimore, 1854), pp. 14-15; *Boston Medical Library, Catalogue of Books in the* . . . (Boston, 1823), pp. iii-iv, listed 619 books.

five dollars and a second of ten dollars.[94] The New York Medical Society offered awards at various times. In 1808 it was a fifty-dollar medal for a paper on topography, geology and mineralogy together with the prevalent diseases in a county, a twenty-five dollar medal for the second choice essay, and another award of twenty-five dollars for the best paper on the causes and cures of typhus.[95] The Medical Society of New York City offered, in 1827, a prize which probably was related to the temperance movement. It was:

Resolved, That this Society will give a premium of fifty dollars, or a medal of the same value, for the best dissertation on the various kinds of beverages in common use, embracing a description of their qualities and of their effects upon health, pointing out particularly such articles as may be substituted for ardent spirits.[96]

By far the largest prize, one of $300, was offered by the Medical Society of Delaware in 1797; but it was not awarded, since no dissertation was deemed worthy by the committee.[97] Although unimportant, these prizes reflect the efforts of the medical groups to encourage writing on medical topics.

It has been said that the medical societies convened and listened to the address of the president or some other member, and then proceeded to the business of regulating the monopoly which the more generous states granted them.

---

[94] Boylston Medical Society. *Act of Incorporation* (Boston, 1853), p. 19.

[95] New York State Medical Society. *Proceedings, 1807-1831*, p. 9.

[96] Medical Society of New York County, *Minutes, 1807-1813*, 1827, p. 354.

[97] *Medical Repository*, I, p. 115. Davis, *Medical Education*, p. 10, credits Delaware with a society in 1776, but I have found no such evidence. Beck, L. P., *The Delaware State Medical Society and its founders in the 18th Century* (New York, 1886), pp. 1 and 4 says that it was organized in 1789 and re-incorporated in 1819. There is statutory evidence of the society of 1819.

MEDICAL REGULATIONS AND SOCIETIES 229

They complained about the irregular, tried to use their corporate influence to improve the education of new doctors and, lastly, awarded occasional prizes for results of study. All this endeavor was related to the doctors' social, professional and financial standing. The social interests of physicians are revealed by participation in reform movements. Rarely did great social changes come from the profession alone, but many doctors, individually and collectively, aided philanthropic and humanitarian activities.

Among these interests was the relation of the apothecary to medical practice. Although the organization of the Philadelphia College of Pharmacy in 1825 was a great aid to the profession, reform of that trade was necessary. Before and after its establishment, however, the medical societies bombarded the legislatures and public with suggestions to prevent the adulteration of drugs. The Connecticut Medical Society tried unsuccessfully to bring about reforms in 1817 and 1822.[98] The same group also recommended that "the apothecaries prepare their medicine according to the Pharmacopoeia of the United States." [99] Much later, the Alabama Convention of 1847 proposed the following: (1) licensing of apothecaries; (2) fining of druggists who prescribed; (3) listing of the ingredients of patent medicines upon the labels.[100] Finally in 1848, the American Medical Association made the proposals which we have previously discussed.[101] Since drugs were largely imported, the Association asked the state societies to petition their congressmen for a law to prevent the adulteration of drugs.[102] In re-

[98] *Connecticut Medical Society, Constitution of* . . . (Hartford, 1824), p. 19; Connecticut Medical Society, *Transactions, 1792-1829*, pp. 193-203.
[99] Connecticut Medical Society, *Transactions, 1792-1829*, 1822, p. 234.
[100] *Alabama, Proceedings of the Medical Convention of the State of* . . . (Mobile, 1848), pp. 9-11.
[101] American Medical Association, *Transactions, 1848*, pp. 297-301.
[102] *Ibid.*, p. 31.

sponse, the Connecticut Medical Society petitioned Congress for the appointment of inspector of drugs,[103] which evidently brought action, for in the next year the Medical Association of South Carolina requested the Secretary of the Treasury to appoint a more efficient inspector for the part of Charleston. In its meeting of 1850 the society was pleased to note that the unsatisfactory inspector had been removed.[104] It would not be extravagant to say that the movement which reached one peak in the Pure Foods and Drugs Act and is now rising again had its inception in these early days.

The temperance movement early enlisted the superficial support of physicians. An appeal in 1829 shows the attitude of the leaders of the movement toward the profession:

and while the members of your profession have almost daily opportunities of witnessing the destructive operation of the present system of drinking, no persons are better qualified to appreciate the measures of reform [nor to adopt them]. It is indeed gratifying to observe the alacrity and decision with which many of the faculty, in various sections of our Union, lend their aid to the advancement of the greatest moral enterprise of the age. A sufficient proof of this is in the fact, that resolutions recommending total abstinence . . . have been passed in ten societies.[105]

While few societies sponsored tee-totalism, almost all endorsed temperance, seeking, as the essay contests show, substitutes for spiritous medicines. The attitude of the profession is best expressed in a series of resolutions of the Massachusetts Medical Society in 1827 to the effect that con-

[103] Connecticut Medical Society, *Transactions, 1848*, p. 8.
[104] Medical Association of South Carolina, *Minutes, 1849-1850*, pp. 50-51.
[105] *Address to Physicians by . . . the New York City Temperance Society* (New York, 1829), pp. 3-4.

stant use of liquor is harmful; that useful as wine is in fever, except during hot weather, water is better; and that malt liquors are the best tonic.[106] Many of the societies condemned the use of ardent spirits and intemperate use of lighter liquors. When A. H. Stevens spoke in 1849, he expressed the admiration of the profession for the work in the temperance cause of Drs. Rush, Sewall and Watts.[107] Evidently the profession favored temperance more for others than for its own members. N. S. Davis tells us that, at the meeting of the American Medical Association in 1849, " the material bounties were provided in great abundance and variety but without the prodigality of expenditure and profusion of strong drink which have since brought these social occasions into much discredit." [108]

Regulation of apothecaries and interest in temperance are only two of the social activities of the profession. Until the American Medical Association was organized with regular committees on Medical Science, Practical Medicine, Surgery, Obstetrics, Education, Medical Literature, Publications, Registration of Births, Marriages and Deaths, Indigenous Medical Botany, and Drainage, there was no regular committee organization of societies.[109] Nevertheless, there was considerable isolated and sporadic activity. The Medical Society of New York City had a committee investigate and report on the manner of still births in the city.[110] During epidemics the medical societies published available informa-

[106] Massachusetts Medical Society, *Medical Papers*, IV, 1827, pp. 4-6.
[107] Stevens, A. H., *The Plea of Humanity in Behalf of Medical Education*, pp. 20-21.
[108] Davis, N. S., *History of the American Medical Association* (Phila., 1855), p. 87.
[109] American Medical Association, *Transactions, 1848*, list of committees in table of contents.
[110] *Medical Society of New York County, Minutes, 1807-1831*, pp. 263-264.

tion. They suggested ways of making vaccination universal; they favored better care of the insane and indigent sick by fostering insane asylums and various dispensaries and hospitals. As a carrier of disease, the water supply of New York City was much discussed in the medical society.[111] Addresses frequently dealt with the filth in American cities, the need of proper sewage disposal, and kindred subjects. If much seemingly fruitless effort is required to attract public attention to any reform, the medical profession certainly aided the cleaning up of American cities. An unusual study of social conditions was an address by Dr. J. C. Green to the Massachusetts Medical Society in 1846, entitled " Factory System in its Hygienic Relations." While stating that conditions were better in America than in England, he condemned the daily average of twelve hours and eighteen minutes as too long.[112]

A summary of the important general medical societies would include those of Massachusetts, New York, Connecticut, New Jersey and a few others. Besides these general groups more specialized societies grew up in the larger cities. Of the many which came and went, the College of Physicians of Philadelphia, the Society for Medical Improvement of Boston and the New York Academy of Medicine achieved national renown. One of the first medical organizations, the College of Physicians of Philadelphia, received a charter in 1789 with such members as John Redman, William Shippen, Jr., Adam Kuhn, John Morgan, Benjamin Rush, Thomas Parke, Caspar Wistar, Jr., and John Gibbon.[113]

[111] *Medical Society of the State of New York, Proceedings of* . . . *1838-1840* (Albany, 1840), App., pp. 11-12; ibid., *1834-1835*, McCall's lecture on the insane poor, pp. 6-8; ibid., *1807-1831*, pp. 449-450.

[112] Massachusetts Medical Society, *Medical Papers*, VI, 1846, pp. 234-235.

[113] *College of Physicians of Philadelphia, Charter, Ordinance, and By-Laws of* . . . (Phila., 1834), Pref.

The Boston Society for Medical Improvement was organized in 1838. Finally, in 1846 the New York Academy of Medicine completed the trio. All three societies were composed of well-known physicians, who desired medical improvement. The New York Academy of Medicine, in fact, owed its inception partly to the realization of the profession that, after practice was thrown open to all in 1844, it must render still greater service to the public.[114] Other societies of specialized interest, but of national scope, were the Society of Medical Superintendents of Lunatic Asylums, which met biyearly after its foundation in the early 1840's, and the National Society of Dental Surgeons organized in 1839.[115]

The medical societies, then, in a discursive manner played their part in the humantarian and public-spirited activities which characterized America after the war of 1812. To credit the profession with the rise of new and better hospitals, with the growth of dispensaries and infirmaries, with the improved condition of the insane and similar activities, which owe their origin to the heightened social consciousness, would be presumptuous. Suffice it to say that the profession, in its societies and magazines offered aid and encouragement to all such endeavors.

[114] Francis, John W., *Old New York* (N. Y., 1858), p. 322. Among the other societies which might be mentioned chronologically were: The Physico-Medical Society of New York City, 1815-1817; the Medical Society of New Orleans, 1818; the Physico-Medical Society of New Orleans, 1820; Kappa Lambda Society of New York City in the early 1820's and which society caused so much trouble; the New York Medical and Surgical Society, 1835, which left four interesting volumes of manuscript records of its cases (in New York Academy of Medicine). It seems to have been the Members of the Medical Association of the New York Dispensary. In 1850 the Ladies Physiological Institute of Boston and Vicinity was chartered. Such charitable societies as the New York Society for the Relief of Widows and Orphans of Medical Men was founded in 1842 and incorporated in 1843.

[115] *American Journal of Dental Science*, I, 1839, p. 178.

DIFFICULTIES OF THE SOCIETIES

The legislatures were not eager to entrench the societies in monopolies. One by one they or the courts rendered the laws against irregulars ineffective. Other obstacles in the path of the profession's efforts to obtain a monopoly were the indifference of its members, its inability to enforce a code of ethics, the quarrelling within societies and the failure to raise necessary funds for current expenses.

Medical societies often passed out of existence soon after their organization. For example, the Medical Society of North Carolina of 1800 and that of Georgia of 1804 seem to have had few, if any, meetings. Other groups, such as the Wisconsin State Medical Society of 1842, are known to us only through the researches of medical scholars.[116] Many of the state societies like the Massachusetts Medical Society were dying at their roots. For example, the Berkshire Medical Association met on March 1, 1821, but the report on by-laws and fees could not be taken up because of the death of the president and the absence of one other committee member.[117] It is best to let Robert Worthington, Secretary to the Society, tell the story as he did to the Massachusetts Medical Society in 1837:

In 1822, *I* was chosen Secy, which office I have been honored with, up to the time of its death—For a great part of the time *seven & eight* were the usual number of *Fellows* present at the various meetings of the Socy—Often the transaction of business was prevented by a want of the requisite number.—Various methods were adopted at different times to induce the *Fellows* in the County, (The whole number, I do not know) to attend the meetings. Efforts were made to induce the *younger* men in the Profession to become Fellows and united with us in sustaining and rendering useful, the regular meetings of the

[116] Toner, J. M., *Medical Biography* (Phila., 1876), p. 47.
[117] Berkshire Medical Association, Minutes.

MEDICAL REGULATIONS AND SOCIETIES 235

Society.—Objections to *Fellow*-ship were that [they paid too much to the parent society. The last quorum of the society was December, 1833. Worthington continued to call meetings until the funds gave out]. I have heretofor, in correspondence with your Secy—given my individual and so far as I knew, the *Society's* view upon the subject of the causes of its dissolution and having now performed the said office of notifying a *Parent*, of the decease of a *child*, I commit the case to your hands, hoping that by timely aid, *other* branches of the family may be saved from premature death.[118]

In this case there had been financial difficulties, but other societies failed because of a lack or lapse of interest. Even so active a group as the Albany Medical Society did not have a quorum in April, July and October of 1836. In both Maine and Tennessee the state society had a most irregular existence, to say nothing of the situation in Illinois and Indiana, where organizations were alternately sponsored and abolished by the state legislatures. Indifference of the members was reflected in their failure to pay dues. Connecticut tried repeatedly to collect them, but as late as 1848 the difficulties of the treasurer handicapped the society.[119]

Lack of professional morale was also a disturbing factor. Physicians who taught in the medical colleges and endorsed patent medicines would not foster the interests of the group at the expense of their own incomes. Whenever new fads, such as Thomsonism or homeopathy appeared, a section of the regular profession deserted allopathy.[120] All the difficulties in this respect have been observed in the discussion of ethics and the attempts to enforce the rules of the societies.

[118] Berkshire Athenaeum, Miscellaneous Papers, Mss.
[119] Connecticut Medical Society, *Transactions*, *1848*, p. 7.
[120] New York Medical Society, *Proceedings* . . . *1841-1845* (Albany, 1845), App., p. 58.

It is doubtful that the lack of professional dignity is so great today as it was then. Competiton was more unscrupulous, the educational and cultural background was more limited and the training necessary for successful practice was decidedly less than is now required.

Besides these troubles, the members of the profession quarrelled. In New York City, where the factions never were reconciled throughout the period, jealousy alone seems to explain the deplorable situation. Certainly envy, probably of the professorial incomes, seems at the root of the quarrel over the College of Physicians and Surgeons of the City of New York in 1826. The third attempt to found a separate medical faculty in that city was made by Hosack and other professors. A knowledge of Hosack's large income and his high social position sufficiently explains the antagonism which he aroused. The quarrel in the medical school was carried to the medical society of New York City and resulted in the defeat of Hosack for the presidency.[121] Again ill-will prompted some physicians to charge the members of the Kappa Lambda Society of New York (which resembled the Boston Society for Medical Improvement) with aiding each other.[122] Finally, and again in New York, the opposition of the representatives of the older colleges forced the state legislature to pass a law to seat Dr. Coventry, the representative of Geneva College.[123] Obviously New York State witnessed more of these affairs than other states, but the fact that it was such a large state and that physicians in other states quarrelled almost as conspicuously attracted unfavorable public comment.

[121] *New York Medical and Physical Journal*, IV, 1827, p. 320.

[122] *Report of the Committee of the Medical Society of the City and County of New York* (New York, 1831), pp. 1-11.

[123] New York Medical Society, *Proceedings* . . . *1834-1835*, p. 39.

THE AMERICAN MEDICAL ASSOCIATION

Lack of interest in the local societies delayed the formation of a national association. The average member of the profession saw little value in a nation-wide organization. Where medical men had any active local groups, they were inclined to guard their time jealously against encroachments of further meetings. Medical schools with low standards feared a loss in their enrollment if they adopted the same regulations as better schools. Until 1846, the obstacles successfully blocked national organization. It was indifference also which prevented the representatives of various groups from meeting every decade after 1820 in order to revise the *United States Pharmacopoeia*. Between 1820 and the meeting in New York in 1846, however, several attempts were made to create a national society. Nathan Smith Davis, chief instigator of the American Medical Association, states: " The first distinct proposition for a national convention emanated from the faculty of the Medical College of Georgia, at Augusta, and was advocated in the columns of the *Southern Medical and Surgical Journal,* published at the same place, as early as 1835." [124] In 1838 the *Boston Medical and Surgical Journal* urged such a society, but it was thought premature by several members of the Massachusetts Massachusetts Medical Society. Despite this opposition, a meeting was held in Boston, over which Governor Everett presided, to discuss the merits of such a measure and " a committee was appointed to consult with the Philosophical Society of Philadelphia." [125] Again, the New Hampshire Medical Society in 1839 proposed a meeting, but this effort failed just as the suggestion of the New York Medical

[124] Davis, *Medical Education, 1776-1876*, p. 57.
[125] *Boston Medical and Surgical Journal*, XVI, p. 368 and XIX, pp. 208-209.

Society for a convention in Philadelphia in 1840 for the same purpose.[126]

Such failures seem only to have spurred Nathan Smith Davis on. The minutes of the New York Medical Society for 1845 give the story:

The following preamble and resolution were presented by Dr. Davis and adopted, and

Drs. Davis, McNaughton, and the Secretary, Dr. Van Buren, were appointed a committee to carry out the proposed measure.

Whereas, It is believed that a National Convention would be conducive to the elevation of the standards of medical education in the United States and

Whereas, There is no mode of accomplishing so desirable an object, without concert of action on the part of the medical societies, colleges, and institutions of all states. Therefore,

Resolved, That the New York State Medical Society earnestly recommend a national convention of delegates from medical societies and colleges in the whole Union—to convene in the city of New York, on the first Tuesday in May, in the year 1846, for the purpose of adopting some concerted action on the subject set forth in the foregoing preamble.[127]

The adoption of this resolution by no means assured the success of the proposed meeting. In New York City itself an attack was made upon the meeting by Martyn Paine of the Medical Faculty of New York University. Reaction outside New York was summarized by the *Boston Medical and Surgical Journal* as follows: "There is some diversity of opinions on the expediency of this measure. An ardent manifestation of interest in the probable deliberations of the

[126] *Ibid.*, XX, p. 177; *American Journal of Medical Sciences*, XIII, p. 264.

[127] New York Medical Society, *Proceedings . . . 1844-1846*, 1845, App., p. 148.

congress, distinguish the resolutions of some state societies: while others look coolly, and even suspiciously." Most of the strong schools. " and Massachusetts, Connecticut and Philadelphia " refused to participate.[128] Philadelphia's refusal was attributed to fear of the medical schools of that city that New York University was using the convention to advertise its medical department, but they were somewhat quieted when Martyn Paine made his attack.[129]

Southern attitude was expressed by Dr. R. D. Arnold of Savannah as favorable. He wrote his cousin that:

On Wednesday night next I start for New York as a delegate from the Georgia Medical Society to the National Medical convention about to be held in N. York on the first Tuesday in May. As it promises to be a very interesting meeting in a professional point of view I thought an absence of two weeks would not be paying too dearly for it, particularly as the Society will pay my traveling expenses.[130]

He used this trip to dine with members of the Philadelphia profession, to attend opera and " without knowing it . . . played a game of five dollar whist, but as soon as [he] was square [he] stopped playing." [131]

When the meeting was called to order, sixteen states and a few colleges were present.[132] Efforts to prevent the formation of a society met defeat, when the Convention decided, with less than half the societies and colleges represented, to remain in session by a vote of seventy-four to two. The first slate of officers were Dr. J. Knight of New Haven (Connecticut evidently having changed its mind), President;

[128] *Boston Medical and Surgical Journal*, XXXIV, pp. 262-263.
[129] Davis, *American Medical Association*, pp. 30-31.
[130] Arnold, *Letters*, pp. 27-28.
[131] *Ibid.*, pp. 29-30.
[132] *American Journal of Medical Sciences*, N. S. XII, 1846, pp. 266-273.

John Bell of Philadelphia and Edward Delafield of New York City as Vice-Presidents; R. D. Arnold, of Savannah, Secretary and Alfred Stillé of Philadelphia, Treasurer. Organization of the society completed, plans were made for its meeting in Philadelphia the following year.[133] At Philadelphia the Convention became the American Medical Association and began its uninterrupted career. By strategic location of meetings in Baltimore in 1848, Boston in 1849 and Cincinnati in 1850 new members from other sections were added to the meager membership. In 1856 its membership totaled between three and four thousand.[134]

In the four years following the convention in New York, state organizations were created or revived in Alabama, Tennessee, Pennsylvania, Georgia, North Carolina, South Carolina, Indiana, Missouri, Illinois and Iowa. These state societies together with the established societies gave the profession concerted action, forums in which medical news could be broadcast, and, by means of delegates to the American Medical Association a national agency through which reforms and ideas could be nationalized.

[133] National Medical Convention, *Proceedings, 1846* (New York, 1846), pp. 15-16.
[134] *Ibid.*, Stewart, *op. cit.*, p. 116.

CHAPTER VIII

Developments in American Medicine, 1783 to 1850

WE have already stated that the revolution in medicine after 1850 was made possible by changes occurring between 1783 and 1850. Static as this period was in its superficial aspects, it contained dynamic elements. The result of these underlying changes was already felt in the 1840's when the contagious nature of puerperal fever and the anesthetic use of ether were discovered. A review of the developments of those years will help explain why even greater changes followed.

By 1850 general practitioners had become familiar with several new means of combating diseases. Unlike the work of Pasteur and Koch, none of these discoveries was fundamental to further change. Few of them were spectacular, but they were cumulative evidence that medical progress was being made. One cannot overlook such discoveries as auscultation by the Frenchman, Laennec (1820), and the curative properties of iodine, powder of cinchona bark, morphia and strychnia.[1] Equally significant were the introduction of ergot into America and the presentation by Oliver Wendell Holmes of his theory concerning the contagious nature of puerperal fever. Jenner's check to smallpox also dates from this period.

Surgery, however, contributed the most exciting discovery —anesthesia. This discovery was the result of experimentation on the part of an increasingly inquisitive profession. The generation immediately after the American Revolution produced excellent general-practitioners with great surgical

[1] *On the Progress of Recent Science*, pp. 1-23.

ability, but specialization in surgery was rare until the period after 1815, when Wright Post, Philip Physick and Valentine Mott became prominent. Their success indicates that they possessed a greater knowledge of anatomy and physiology than their predecessors.

In still another field—the treatment of the insane—medical practice made a distinct advance. Although Benjamin Rush had raised his voice in behalf of these unfortunates, it was not until 1830 that moral treatment, which had been introduced a decade earlier, was widely used. Thereafter more and more insane patients were cared for in new hospitals, situated in the country, where they were treated with kindness and were given agreeable work to do. This change is a further example of the profession's willingness to accept new procedures.

But the continuing characteristic of medical practice during these years was reliance upon old methods and remedies. Bloodletting, emetics, purging, sweating, blisters and the common drugs remained well entrenched. The obvious explanation for their persistence was that offered by Jacob Bigelow. In his address on *Self-Limited Diseases*, he stressed the failure of the profession to increase its knowledge of therapy. Great progress had been made in the diagnosis of human ailments, but therapeutic changes had not immediately followed.[2] As long as the actual nature of disease was not clearly understood, old methods would persist. Nevertheless, attacks were made upon prevailing practices. After 1830, diet (especially vegetable diet) and physical education received much consideration both within and without the profession.

Quacks and other irregulars attacked customary medical practices, offering vegetable substitutes and other innocuous remedies. Their attacks made the profession self-conscious;

---

[2] *Cf. supra*, Chapter VII, p. 220.

and their success in breaking down the monopolies granted by state legislatures forced the profession to defend itself by better therapy. Although not a quack, Hahnemann, the founder of homeopathy, was not in the regular profession. He advocated the doctrine that disease can be cured by medicines which cause in a healthy person symptoms similar to those caused by the disease itself. Given in minute doses, such medicines are supposed to cure in inverse ratio to the amount administered.[3] This system, introduced into America in 1825 by Johannis B. Gram in Boston, made great progress.[4] By 1850 its practitioners were very successful and had established a college in Philadelphia. Despite some of the vagaries of its practice, its emphasis upon small doses of medicine and a light diet had a profound effect upon medical practices. Regular doctors, or allopaths, could accept its successful remedies and methods while rejecting the absurd. In this way homeopathy ultimately lost its merit as an unique medical procedure.

It is now possible to trace the changes which account for general improvement of the medical profession. Undoubtedly, education played an important part. In 1800 only four medical colleges existed in America. Slowly at first, and then very rapidly, educational facilities were extended throughout the country. By 1850, every large city had at least one medical school and every state had one or more so situated as to provide education for all students of medicine. Probably such early physicians as Rush, Morgan, Bard or Warren were as well-educated as those who later became renowned, yet few, if any, practitioners of 1850 would have been so illiterate as to write a letter like that quoted in our

[3] *American Journal of Homeopathy* (1 volume, 1838-1839, Phila., 1838-1839), pp. 1-7.
[4] Wilder, A., *History of Medicine*, pp. 316-317.

early pages.[5] It was this general raising of standards which helps explain the fundamental contribution of education to medical change.

The quality of work in our medical schools, likewise, improved. The terms were lengthened from twelve, thirteen and fourteen weeks to sixteen, twenty and even twenty-four weeks. In addition, schools made use of short courses, reading terms and anatomical laboratories to give students additional opportunities. In the years which we are discussing the average number of professorships was increased from three to seven. This increase meant a corresponding specialization on the part of professors, a factor conducive to better education. General requirements, also, rose during these years. Those dealing with practical anatomy and hospital attendance were particularly important. It is doubtful whether there was any member of the profession of 1850 who had never seen "the inside of a corpse." Naturally with more stringent requirements, better facilities were supplied. The students' laboratories were generally better arranged than those of earlier years. Meager as they were, the libraries were larger and contained better selected references.

In another respect, the student, both in and out of college, had an additional advantage. New and superior textbooks were coming from the presses. In anatomy, illustrations became a definite part of a satisfactory text. In all fields the tempo of publication quickened; this trend meant not only a faster turnover in textbooks, but also the production of better organized texts with the latest information. By 1850 textbooks written fifty or even seventy-five years earlier, were not in use—because the profession was more alert and also because scientific changes demanded more frequent revision. One does not have to be a chauvinist to value the fact that,

[5] *Cf. supra*, Chapter I, pp. 19-20.

by 1850, the percentage of these books written by Americans was greater than it had been at the beginning of the period.

After the establishment of the *American Medical Repository,* the number of magazines increased until twenty-four circulated throughout the country. Almost all these were superior to the early publications. In the first place, they represented a change from the days when physicians had to report their interests in general philosophical or scientific journals. Secondly, they were better edited and published. Thirdly, they were more scientific and less discursive. Fourthly, some of the articles attracted attention outside America; thus many articles by Professor Jackson were transcribed to European journals.[6] Finally, the medical journals served the entire nation.

Besides the magazines, societies increased in number and influence. Few and unimportant in the early years, they multiplied until they were available to the entire profession. In the states and cities they made possible numerous contacts among physicians and brought together delegates from various districts. Oddly enough, medical laws, though an impetus to the formation of societies, were repealed just at the time when the professional monopoly was beginning to produce desired results. From the point of view of the societies this loss of power was not so important, for they were then organized and could proceed with their professional interests. Out of the state organizations grew the American Medical Association. At the time of its appearance, the scientific movement was coming into its own; and this national society provided a central body to judge education, to evaluate innovations in the various phases of medicine and to give the profession a sense of concerted action.

Thus far we have looked for changes in the doctor's background—in his medical practices, his education, in his books,

[6] *Cf. supra,* Chapter VI, p. 197.

magazines and societies. There were in addition, forces cutting across these fields as well as factors which indirectly affected the medical profession. The most significant of these was the trend toward specialization. As any branch of knowledge becomes complex, it is impossible for an individual to master it; specialization logically follows. As a result, new discoveries are made, and complexity increases. In the case of medicine contributing factors were the growth of cities, where doctors mastered one phase of medicine in order to serve a small group, and the increased enrollments in colleges which required a larger faculty. Specialization did not begin in one section of the nation or one phase of medicine and then spread to others; it was an interacting development. In education, the number of professorships not only increased, but professors did not move from one chair to another. In the early medical schools a professor in the course of his life might teach all subjects in the curriculum. This situation undoubtedly created well-rounded physicians, such as Rush. He did so many things, however, that he never carried one interest to its end. For instance, if he had stressed his ideas on the treatment of the insane, he might have reformed American conditions during his lifetime. It is significant that, despite Rush's amazing discoveries (many of which are known only to research men), he was famous for his use of bloodletting and calomel, both of which practices failed to survive the test of time. As a specialist in a chosen field on the other hand, he would have been less likely to lose sight of valuable changes in method.

In the practice of medicine, this tendency toward specialization led to the separation of dentistry from surgery. It was probably not pure chance that prompted a dentist to ask a regular physician for some means of deadening pain, with the result that Dr. Jackson mentioned the anesthetic possibilities of ether to Dr. Morton. As time passed, surgery, in the larger cities, became separated from general practice. Even midwifery, in Philadelphia, had such authorities as Dewees and Meigs, the latter's reputation in diseases of women prompting Dr. Arnold to send his wife from Savannah to Philadelphia for treatment.

In the care of the insane, we find the same development. We have referred to Benjamin Rush's proposals for improvement of such treatment. Subsequently, there appeared a group of specialists in the care of the insane. Ultimately, they had their own society and magazine. From their reports and discussions, a body of information on the care of patients became available. By 1850 their combined experience made possible the publication of standards for a good asylum.

Not only in education and practice but in the publication of magazines and the organization of societies the same trend toward specialization appeared. In 1797 the only medical magazine was a *repository*. At that time the profession had to rely upon sympathetic philosophical and scientific journals for publication, but by 1850 it had magazines which covered general medicine, medical bibliography, dentistry and insanity. The larger cities had their special societies, and the committees of the American Medical Association sharply differentiated the various fields of medicine. In addition to these groups, there arose other societies with such interests as insanity and dentistry, their establishment reflecting the growth of specialization.

Various developments within the nation itself were affecting medical history. During the years from 1783 to 1850, the United States made great material advances, so that by the latter date, the nation could support many institutions which colonial society could not have afforded. Furthermore, after the conquest of a vast section of wilderness, men turned from these struggles with nature itself to devote more of their time and money to their cultural interests. More wealth was available for academies and colleges, for hospitals and asylums. With the growth of these institutions, medicine and the medical profession were profoundly affected. No longer were Americans so completely dependent upon Europe. Their increasing self-reliance was revealed in various ways—in their use of medical textbooks written by their own countrymen, in their publications which supplanted European works, and in their ability to state and to test new scientific hypotheses.

Both American and European medicine profited from movements not necessarily part of medicine. By 1800, science, no longer an amusing plaything, had become a valuable instrument. Chemistry was making great progress in the discovery of methods and elements; thus we have seen that chemical analysis filled a much larger section of books on chemistry in 1850 than in earlier years.[7] General scientific interest looked to the new with hope rather than suspicion; such a popular attitude made the introduction of new methods and remedies much easier. This scientific interest created within the profession itself a faculty of observation far keener than that possessed by men of similar ability in the early part of this period.

Two other developments profoundly affected medical progress; cheap publication and new means of communication and transportation. We have traced the history of magazines and noted their influence upon practitioners. Undoubtedly such men as Rush and his Philadelphia colleagues would have liked to publish a medical journal, but such an undertaking was more expensive than the size of the country or the interest of the profession would warrant. If publishing had not become cheaper, it is very doubtful whether the profession of 1850 could have supported twenty-four medical periodicals.

[7] *Cf. supra*, Chapter III, p. 69.

The spread of information is, of course, dependent upon means of communication. As these facilities increased, the physicians throughout the nation were brought into closer contact with each other. Professional solidarity grew. American physicians could go to Europe, or could receive the latest European journals. The world was brought closer together; and although we are here treating the American phase of medical history, it must be remembered that much of American practice, often the better portion, had come from Europe. From it we obtained vaccination, auscultation, such drugs as ergot and iodine, and not a few of our textbooks. While, in 1850, we were writing quite a number of our own texts, those from England and the Continent reached us soon after publication. From this inter-dependence and inter-relation of the two continents, medicine could be expected to acquire new and better methods.

By the middle of the century, then, various changes had quietly brought medicine to the verge of a revolution. Practices were not dissimilar from those of an earlier age, but confidence in them had been undermined, and the way was prepared for a series of discoveries which has continued to the present day. Alert individuals sensed this impending change. It is not surprising, therefore, to hear Samuel Gross exclaim:

It requires no prophetic eye, no special forecast, to discover that we are on the very verge of one of the most fearful and wide-spread revolutions in medicine that the world has ever witnessed; another of those astounding changes whose name is already legion, and which, whether for good or evil, is destined to convulse the profession, and to exert a most powerful influence upon the practice of the healing art.[8]

[8] Gross, S. D., *Brunonianism, Toddism, and Otherism* (Phila., 1861), p. 5.

BIBLIOGRAPHICAL NOTE

The sources upon which this study of the medical profession is based are varied and widely scattered. Fortunately, the *Index-Catalogue of the Library of the Surgeon-General's Office, United States Army* (16 volumes, Washington, 1880-1895; Second Series, 21 volumes, Washington, 1896-1916; and, the Third Series, 10 volumes, Washington, 1918-1932) supplies an excellent guide to the printed materials. Although there are a number of general books on the history of medicine which partly cover the period from 1783 to 1850, the following have been most helpful: F. H. Garrison, *An Introduction to the History of Medicine* (Philadelphia and London, 1917), for an excellent background of medical history; F. R. Packard, *History of Medicine in the United States* (2 volumes, New York, 1931), which contains much valuable information and is a useful guide to further study; H. E. Sigerist, *American Medicine* (New York, 1834), (Translated from the German by Hildegard Nagel); Walter L. Burrage, *A History of the Massachusetts Medical Society... 1781-1922* (Boston, 1923); James Joseph Walsh, *History of Medicine in New York*... (5 volumes, New York, 1919); *History of the Medical Society of the District of Columbia . . . 1817-1909* (Washington, 1909); N. S. Davis, *Contributions to the History of the Medical Education and Medical Institutions in the United States, 1776-1876* (Washington, 1877); T. F. Harrington, *The Harvard Medical School. A History, Narrative and Documentary, 1782-1905* (3 volumes, New York and Chicago, 1905); *The University of Pennsylvania* (Phila., 1841); S. D. Gross, *American Medical Literature* (Philadelphia, 1876); and, S. D. Gross, Ed., *Lives of Eminent American Physicians and Surgeons of the 19th Century* (Philadelphia, 1861).

Much of the primary source material has been discussed in the text. Chapter III, for example, contains information on the medical textbooks which have been consulted. The most important laws regulating the practice of medicine, have been fully cited in the footnote references for Chapter VII. The pamphlets, of which there are many, have been listed in the footnotes, particularly for Chapters V and VII.

This bibliographical note, then, is limited to a list of the more useful magazines, the transactions of the medical societies, catalogs or circulars of the colleges and the account books and similar materials of physicians.

MEDICAL MAGAZINES

American (The) Journal of Dental Science (10 volumes, New York, Baltimore, Boston and Philadelphia, 1839-1850).
American Journal of Insanity (6 volumes, Utica, New York, 1844-1850).
American (The) Journal of the Medical Sciences (26 volumes, Philadelphia, 1827-1840; N. S. 18 volumes, Philadelphia, 1841-1850). Continuation of: *Philadelphia Journal of Medical and Physical Sciences.*
American (The) Medical Recorder (6 volumes, Philadelphia, 1818-1823). Continued as: *Medical (The) Recorder of Original Papers.*
American (The) Medical Repository (24 volumes, New York, 1797-1824).
Boston Medical Intelligencer (5 volumes, Boston, 1822-1826). United with *New England Journal of Medicine and Surgery* to form:
Boston Medical and Surgical Journal (40 volumes, Boston, 1828-1850).
Illinois (The) Medical and Surgical Journal (2 volumes, Chicago, 1844-1846). Continued as:
Illinois and Indiana Medical and Surgical Journal (2 volumes, Chicago and Indianapolis, 1846-1848). Continued as:
Northwestern Medical and Surgical Journal (beginning with Volume v, volumes v to vii, Chicago and Indianapolis, 1848-1850).
Journal of Foreign Medical Science and Literature (4 volumes, Philadelphia, 1821-1824). Merged in 1825 with: *American (The) Medical Recorder.*
Journal of the Philadelphia College of Pharmacy (Old series, 1 volume, numbers 1-4, Philadelphia, 1825-1827; N. S. 6 volumes, Philadelphia, 1829-1835). In 1835, merged with: *American Journal of Pharmacy* (18 volumes, Philadelphia, 1835-1852).
Medical News and Library (8 volumes, Philadelphia, 1843-1850).
Missouri (The) Medical and Surgical Journal (4 volumes, St. Louis, 1845-1848). Merged with: *Saint Louis Medical and Surgical Journal.*
New England Quarterly Journal of Medicine and Surgery (1 volume, Boston, 1842-1843).
New Orleans Medical Journal (1 volume, New Orleans, 1844-1845). In July, 1845, it united with the *Louisiana Medical and Surgical Journal* to form:
New Orleans (The) Medical and Surgical Journal (Volumes ii-vi, New Orleans, 1845-1850).
New England Journal of Medicine and Surgery (15 volumes, Boston, 1812-1826). United with the *Boston Medical Intelligencer* to form the *Boston Medical and Surgical Journal.*
New York (The) Journal of Medicine and Collateral Sciences (9 volumes, New York, 1843-1848; N. S. 16 volumes, New York, 1848-1856).
New York Medical and Philosophical Journal and Review (3 volumes, New York, 1809-1811).

New-York Medical and Physical Journal (9 volumes, New York, 1822-1830).
North American Medical and Surgical Journal (12 volumes, Philadelphia, 1826-1831).
Ohio Medical and Surgical Journal (3 volumes, Columbus, 1848-1850).
Philadelphia Journal of Medical and Physical Sciences (9 volumes, Philadelphia, 1820-1824; N. S. 5 volumes, Philadelphia, 1825-1827). Continued as: *American Journal of the Medical Sciences.*
Philadelphia Medical and Physical Journal (3 volumes, Philadelphia, 1804-1809).
Philadelphia Medical Museum (6 volumes, Philadelphia, 1804-1811).
Saint Louis Medical and Surgical Journal (8 volumes, St. Louis, 1843-1850). In September 1848, number 2 of volume VI, *The Missouri Medical and Surgical Journal* merged with this journal.
Select (The) Medical Library and Eclectic Journal of Medicine (4 volumes, Philadelphia, 1836-1840). Continued as:
Select (The) Medical Library and Bulletin of Medical Science (N. S. 6 volumes, Philadelphia, 1841-1846).
Southern (The) Medical and Surgical Journal (3 volumes, Augusta, Georgia, 1826-1839; N. S., 17 volumes, Augusta, 1845-1861).
Transylvania (The) Journal of Medicine and the Associated Sciences (12 volumes, Lexington, Kentucky, 1828-1839).
Western (The) Journal of Medicine and Surgery (8 volumes, Louisville, 1840-1843; 2nd series, 8 volumes, Louisville, 1844-1847; 3rd series, 6 volumes, Louisville, 1848-1850).
Woods Quarterly Retrospect of American and Foreign Practical Medicine and Surgery (2 volumes, New York, 1847-1849).

TRANSACTIONS OF THE MEDICAL SOCIETIES

Albany, Annals of the Medical Society of the County of . . . Ed. Sylvester D. Willard (Albany, 1851).
American Medical Association, Transactions of the . . . (3 volumes, Philadelphia, 1848-1850).
Association of the Medical Superintendents of American Institutions for the Insane, History of the . . . John Curwen (Warren, Pennsylvania, 1885) (Since this is practically an edition of the minutes, it is placed here).
Connecticut Medical Society, 1792-1829, Transactions of the . . . (Hartford, 1884).
Connecticut Medical Society, Proceedings at the Annual Convention of the . . . (Hartford, 1791-1850).
Medical and Chirurgical Faculty of Maryland, Transactions of the . . . (Baltimore, 1799-1850).

BIBLIOGRAPHY

Massachusetts Medical Society, Medical Papers Communicated to the . . . (Boston, 1790-1850).
National Medical Convention, Minutes of the proceedings of the . . . *1846* (New York, 1846).
New Hampshire Medical Society, Records of the . . . *from its organization in 1791 to the year 1854* (Concord, 1911).
New Jersey Medical Society, The Rise, Minutes, and Proceedings of the . . . *Established July 23rd, 1766* (Newark, 1875).
New York Academy of Medicine, Transactions of the . . . (New York, 1847-1851).
New York, Minutes of the Medical Society of the City and County of . . . *1807-1831* (New York, 1831).
New York State Medical Society, Transactions of the . . . *1806-1831* (Albany, 1869).
New York State Medical Society, Transactions of the . . . (Various places, 1827-1850).
Ohio, Proceedings of the Convention of Physicians of . . . (Columbus, 1835-1850).
Philadelphia, Transactions of the College of Physicians of . . . (Philadelphia, 1790-1850).
Tennessee, Transactions and Proceedings of the Medical Society of the State of . . . (Nashville, 1830-1850).

COLLEGE CATALOGS

The following is a list of the colleges and the years for which their catalogs, circulars or announcements, whatever their current name might be, have been used. The list begins with the New York Regent's report since that item includes: the Albany Medical College, Columbia Medical College, the College of Physicians and Surgeons of New York City (with the exceptions of 1834, 1835, 1836 and 1837), the College of Physicians and Surgeons of the Western District, Geneva Medical College and the Medical Department of the University of the City of New York.

New York State, *Senate Journal*, 1791, 1792, Nov. 1792, 1795, 1796, Nov. 1796, 1802, 1803, 1805, 1806, 1807, 1808, 1816, 1818, 1820, 1823, 1824, 1825 and 1827 (Albany, 1791-1827). All dates are January unless otherwise noted.

———, *Assembly Journal*, 1794, 1798, 1800, Nov. 1800, 1904, 1809, 1810, 1811, 1812, 1813, 1814, 1815, 1816, 1819, 1821, 1822 and 1826 (Albany, 1794-1826). All dates are January unless otherwise noted.

———, *Documents*, 1830, III; 1831, I; 1834, II; 1846, II (Albany, 1830-1846). All dates are January.

University of the State of New York, *Annual Reports of the Regents, 1827-1850* (Albany, 1827-1850).

BIBLIOGRAPHY

Albany Medical College, 1838-1850.
Berkshire Medical School, 1822-1824, 1826, 1828-1831, 1835, 1837, 1839-1842, 1845-1848.
Medical School of Maine (Bowdoin), 1823, 1826, 1828-1829, 1833, 1835-1838, 1840-1843, 1849.
University of Buffalo, 1846-1850.
Castleton Medical College, 1822-1825, 1827-1837, 1840-1850.
Cincinnati College, Medical Department of . . . 1835-1838, 1845.
Columbian Medical College, 1841-1842, 1844-1846, 1848, 1849.
Dartmouth College (New Hampshire Medical School), 1829, 1844, 1845, 1848, 1849, 1850.
Evansville Medical College, 1850-1851.
Female Medical College of Pennsylvania, 1853-1854.
Franklin Medical College, 1849.
Geneva Medical College, 1842, 1844, 1845.
Georgia, Medical College of . . . , 1847-1848.
Harvard University, Medical School of . . . , 1836-1837, 1840-1841 to 1849-1850.
Homeopathic Medical College of Pennsylvania, 1848-1881.
Illinois College, Jacksonville, 1846-1847.
Indiana Medical College, LaPorte, 1842-1843, 1845-1846, 1846-1847, 1849-1850.
Jefferson Medical College, 1832, 1835, 1837-1840, 1843, 1845-1846.
Louisville, University of . . . , 1837-1838 to 1841-1842; 1844-1845 to 1853-1854.
Maryland, University of . . . Alumni of the school of medicine, 1813-1850. Catalogs, etc., 1839-1840 to 1841-1842; 1844-1845 to 1846-1847, 1848.
Medical Department of Kemper College, 1842.
Memphis Institute, 1849-1850.
Michigan, Medical Department of the University of . . . , 1850.
Missouri Medical College, St. Louis, 1840-1841 to 1846-1847, 1848-1849, 1850-1851.
Nashville, Medical Department of the University of . . . , 1851-1852.
New England Female Medical College, Boston, 1848-1850.
New York, Medical Department of the University of the City of . . . , 1841, 1842, 1843-1850.
New York, College of Physicians and Surgeons in the City of . . . , 1828-1829, 1836-1837 to 1850-1851.
Ohio, Medical College of . . . , 1829-1830, 1834, 1835-1836, 1836-1837, 1841-1842 to 1850-1851.
Pennsylvania, Medical Department of the University of . . . , 1836, 1843, 1846, 1850.
Philadelphia College of Medicine, 1847-1850.

BIBLIOGRAPHY

Rush Medical College, 1849-1850.
Rutgers Medical College, 1827, 1828-1830.
St. Louis Medical College, 1844-1845, 1847-1848, 1849-1850.
South Carolina, Medical College of . . . , 1837-1838.
South Carolina, Medical College of the State of . . . , 1835-1836 to 1837-1838, 1841, 1844-1845 to 1849-1850.
Starling Medical College, 1847-1848, 1848-1849, 1849-1850.
Transylvania, School of Dental Surgery of . . . , 1850-1851.
Tremont Street Medical School in Boston, 1847-1849.
Upper Mississippi, College of Physicians and Surgeons of the . . . , 1849-1850.
Vermont Medical College, 1835-1850.
Vermont, Medical Department of the University of . . . , 1823-1836.
Virginia, University of . . . , 1825-1843, 1844-1845, 1846-1848, 1849-1850.
Washington University of Baltimore, 1841-1842, 1843-1844 to 1845-1846, 1847-1848.
Western District, College of Physicians and Surgeons of the . . . , 1823-1824, 1836-1837 to 1850-1851.
Western Reserve University, 1846-1847, 1848-1849.
Willoughby University, Medical Department of . . . , 1839-1840, 1841-1842, 1845-1846.
Yale College, 1826-1827 to 1856.

Manuscripts

The following is a list of the Account Books, Day Books and other record books together with the Libraries in which they are kept.

Berkshire Athenaeum, Pittsfield, Massachusetts.
    Childs, Henry H., Letters.
    Childs, Timothy, Day Book 1813-1834.
Boston Medical Library, Boston, Massachusetts.
    Adams, Charles G., Ledger, September, 1824-1834.
    Adams, Daniel, Account Book, 1810-1818.
    Aspinwell, William, Account Book, 1791-1797.
    Bigelow, Jacob, Ledger, 1837-1846.
    Fox, George, Wallingford, Vermont, Day Book, 1809.
    Lloyd, James, Ledger, 1782-1810.
    Pierce, Daniel, Ledger, 1791-1800.
    Pierson, A. L., Letter Book, 1823-1828.
    Post, Minturn, Philadelphia, Diary, 1830-1861.
    Shattuck, G. C., Account Books, 1824-1842.
    Shattuck, G. C., Journal, 1833-1836.
    Shattuck, G. C., Notebook, 1836.
    Shattuck, G. C., Jr., Diary, 1829-1849.

BIBLIOGRAPHY

  Spofford, Richard S., Newburyport, Massachusetts, Account Books, 1828-1829, 1840-1845.
  Strong, Woodbridge, Account Book, 1818-1819.
  Sweat, William, Hollis, New Hampshire, Day Book, No. 13, Nov. 1st, 1825 to Sept. 11, 1831.
  Thaxter, Thomas, Account Book, 1793-1809.
  Warren, John, Sr., Day Book, 1781-1791.
  Whitney, Isaiah, Ledger, 1823-1827.
  Author unknown, Recipe Book, 1812-1813.
  Author unknown, Journal of Practice, 1817.
  Author unknown, Journal from August 28th, 1830 to July 18, 1831.
Hunterdon County Historical Society, Flemington, New Jersey.
  Bowne, John, Account Books, 1801-1807.
Massachusetts Historical Society, Boston, Massachusetts.
  Warren, John, Sr., Day Books.
New Jersey Historical Society, Newark, New Jersey.
  Kunz and Hayes, Day-Books, 1819-1828.
  Sweet and Robinson, Account Books, 1858-1866.
  Turk, William, Journal, U. S. Surgeon.
New York Academy of Medicine.
  Hanford, David, Day Book, 1816-1842.
  Hosack, David, Letters, 1807-1816.
  Phinny, Dr. Sturgis, Day-Book, 1821-1825.
New York Public Library.
  Gansevoort Papers.
  Frances Papers.
New York State Library, Albany, New York.
  Frary, Robert, Day-Book, 1822-1838.
Pennsylvania Historical Society, Philadelphia, Pennsylvania.
  Bache Papers.
  Bond, Dr. Phineas, Receipt Book, 1759-1810.
  Dreer Collection of Letters of Physicians, Surgeons and Chemists.
  Etting Collection, Physicians.
  Gratz Collection.
  Johnston Collection, 1824.
  Peters Manuscripts.
  Wallace Papers.
The Day Books of Dr. Henry Pleasants for 1815 at Hamiltonville, Pennsylvania and Hamilton Village, 1834, have been used through the kind permission of the present Dr. Henry Pleasants, of Westchester, Pennsylvania.

Fee-tables

The following is a complete list of the fee-tables which have been used:

Belmont (Ohio) Medical Society, 1847.
Berkshire Medical Association, 1821.
Boston, May, 1782, 1788, 1806 and 1817.
Buffalo, 1830 and 1836.
Charleston, 1792, 1804 and 1850.
College of Physicians, Philadelphia, 1789 and 1834.
Hampden District Medical Society, Massachusetts, 1858.
Hartford, Connecticut, 1831.
Kentucky, 1841.
King's County, New York, 1835.
Louisiana and Mississippi, 1843.
Lowell Medical Association, Massachusetts, 1837.
Maryland, 1854.
New Jersey, 1766.
New York City, 1790, 1798 and 1816.
Niagara County, New York, Rates for the poor, 1841-1843.
Washington, D. C., 1837.
Washington County, New York, 1838.

INDEX

Abortion, 135; grounds for expulsion from a medical society, 222
Advertising, rates in magazines, 189; patent medicine, 203; grounds for expulsion from a medical society, 222
Alabama (State of), medical regulations, 212, 240
Alabama Medical Convention, 52; proposals for regulating apothecaries and patent medicine, 229
Albany Medical College, established, 40; state appropriation and city endowment, 45; library, 73
Albany, Medical Society of, 211 n. 37; enforcement of medical ethics, 221-223; library, 226; irregularity of meetings, 235
Alcott, W. A., works, 180-181
American Academy of Arts and Sciences (Boston), 23
American Annals of the Deaf and Dumb, 185
American Journal of Dental Science, 184
American Journal of Insanity, 185
American Journal of the Medical Sciences, 183; book reviews, 193
American Medical Association, relation to medical education, 42; report on term of study, 51-52; educational reform, 78; proposal for educational reform, 93-94; rôle in educational reform, 95; ethics, 148; on the editing of British writings, 178; remarks on advertising in the magazines, 190; criticism of magazines, 199; report on medical regulation, 214; attempts to improve quality of drugs, 229-230; drinking at meetings of, 231; committees, 231; account of, 237-240
American Medical Repository: see *Medical Repository*
American Museum, 21, 22

American Philosophical Society, 23; honors to physicians, 170
Amputation, 139
Anatomy, Shippin's work, 14, 16; fees for courses, 48; laboratory fees, 49; laboratories, 52; study of, 56-67
Anesthesia, 11, 24, 138, 140-145, 241-242
Anthelmintics, 103
Apothecaries, Percival's attitude toward and ethics, 152; regulation in Louisiana, 212; attempts to regulate, 229
Apprenticeship, 19; charges, 33-34, 54
Arkansas (State of), lack of medical legislation, 214
Arnold, R. D., treatment of Cholera Asiatic in the South, 114; on feminine modesty, 130; income, 168; lack of southern medical writing, 178; delegate to American Medical Association, 239; Secretary of American Medical Association, 240
Arteriotomy, 97
Ashburn, P. M., list of public officials who were physicians, 171
Asthma, treatment of, 108
Athens, Plague of, compared with yellow fever, 111
Auscultation, 241
Awl, W. A., 129

Bache, B. Franklin and Wood, G. B., 72
Bachelor of Medicine degree, 15, 36; discontinued at the University of Pennsylvania, 74
Baillie, M., 62
Baltimore, anatomical riots, 58
Baltimore Medical and Physical Recorder, 182
Baltimore Medical Society, 22
Baltimore Medical and Surgical Journal and Review, 183

INDEX

Barclay, J., 62
Bard, John, 22, 26
Bard, Samuel, 26, 78; educational ideas, 90, 171
Barter, 164-165
Bartlett, John, 171
Bartlett, J. S., quarrel with the Massachusetts Medical Society, 223-224
Bartlett, Josiah, vaccination, 110-111
Barton, B. S., author, 174
Barton, W. P. C., 72
Bayle, O. L., 63
Beaumont, Wm., *Physiology of Digestion*, 68
Beck, J. B., 72; rules for administering anesthesia, 142-143
Beck, T. R., 72, 171
Beck, Wendell and Ludlow, report on terms of study, 51-52
Bedford, G. S., 85
Bell, Sir Charles, 62, 63, 65
Bell, John (of Philadelphia), Vice-President of the American Medical Association, 240
Bell, John, 62, 63
Bennett, Jesse, 135, n. 120
Berkshire Medical Association, petition for medical college, 225; account of, 234-235
Berkshire Medical College, established, 39; state appropriation, 46; fees, 48; boarding house rates, 50; reading term, 53; condemned for "body-snatching," 59; rowdy spirit, 76; farewell party to graduates, 77; hospital attendance of pupils, 89
Bichat, Xavier, 62-63, 67
Bigelow, Jacob, 72; "Discourse on Self-Limited Diseases," 220
Bigelow, Jacob, Jr., European study, 43, 165
Blackwell, Elizabeth, 37; health education, 179-180
Blackwell's Island, hospital for the insane, 119
Bleecher, Hermanus, 83
Blisters, 101
Bloodletting, 23, 26; Sydenham's use of, 29, 96-99
Bloomingdale Hospital for the insane, 119; lectures, 125
Blumenbach, J. F., 63
Blundell, J., 72

Boards (Medical), 211-213
Board and room expenses, 50
Boardman, Andrew, criticism of Geneva College, 90
Boerhaave, Herman, theory of, 25, 26, 70
Book reviews, 193-195
Boston, hospital for the insane, 119; medical fees, 156-158 ff; homeopathy introduced, 243
Boston Medical Association, medical fees, 157-158
Boston Medical Intelligencer, 182; asserts its independence, 188
Boston Medical Library, 23
Boston Medical Police, 148
Boston Medical Society, fees, 156
Boston Medical and Surgical Journal, 182; on profits from medical magazines, 188; support of national medical society, 237
Boston Society of Medical Improvement, Holmes's lecture on puerperal fever, 136, 232-233
Botanic medicines, use at Memphis Medical Institute, 41, 201-202, 213
Botany, 14
Bowdoin College (Maine Medical College), established, 39; fees, 48, 86; educational reform, 92
Boylston Medical Society, 227-228
Brigham, Amariah, 125-126; income, 169
Brown, John, 25
Brown University, Medical Department of, established, 39
Buffalo, Medical Department of the University of, established, 41; library, 73
Buffalo Medical Journal, 184
Burns, T., 72
Butler Asylum, 129

Cadavers, advertised price at Geneva College, 90
Cadwalader, Thomas, 56
Cæsarian section, 135 and n. 120
Caldwell, Charles, remark on Philadelphia magazines, 193-194
Calomel, 99
Carolina Journal of Medicine, Science and Agriculture, 183
Carus, C. G., 63
Castleton Medical School (Vermont), established, 39; term of

INDEX

study, 51; two terms, 54; anatomical riot, 59, 85-86
Cathartics, 99-100
Chamberlen, Hugh, instruments for midwifery, 134
Channing, Walter, use of ether, 144
Chapman, Nathaniel, 71; treatment of constipation, 104-105
Charity Hospital (New Orleans), insane department, 117
Charleston Medical Journal and Review, 185
Charleston Medical Register, 182
Charleston Medical Society, 22-23
Chemistry, in Morgan's plan for education, 14; Rush professor of, 26; fees for course, 48; study of, 68-69; 69 n. 41; improvements, 248
Cheselden, W., 62
Chicago, number of physicians, 166
Cholera Asiatic, treatment of, 112-114, 184; laws of New York and Rhode Island during epidemic of, 217
Cholera Bulletin, 184
Cholera Gazette, 184
Cholera Infantum, treatment of, 114
Christian tradition, factor in history of midwifery, 130
Church, Benjamin, 27
Cincinnati, Commercial Hospital, 81; Eye Infirmary, 81; number of physicians, 166
Cincinnati, Med. College of, closes temporarily, 41; Drake at, 79
Clergy, censure by medical societies for endorsement of patent medicines, 225
Clinical lectures, fees for, 50
Cloquet, H., 63
Cobbett, William, quarrel with Benjamin Rush, 31
Colden, Cadwalader, 21
Colleges (Medical), 13, 17-19, 38-41, 42
Columbia University (Medical College), 17-19; publication of theses, 75; attempt to form graduate school, 77
Columbian Medical College, established, 40; closes temporarily, 41; fees, 48; aid to poor, 48, 75-76
Commercial Hospital (Cincinnati), 81

Congress, Rush's protest against army-hospital conditions, 28; law permitting sentence of dissection, 60
Connecticut, laws permitting dissection, 60, 61; insane asylum, 119; regulations of medical practice, 208-209
Connecticut Medical Society, established, 22; control of education, 44; regulation of medical practice, 208-209; 218-240, *passim*
Constipation, treatment of, 104-105
Constitution, 21, 27
Contagion, in yellow fever, 1-11; in puerperal fever, 136
Contributors to medical magazines, 187-188
Conway Cabal, Rush and, 27, 28
Cooper, Sir Astley and Samuel, 69, 138
Copeland, Thomas, weaning, 137
Croup, 107-108
Cruvelhier, H., 63
Cullen, William, theories, 14, 25; teacher of Rush, 26, 27; Rush rejects theories of, 29, 67, 70
Cupping, 97
Curriculum, Morgan's plan, 14; development, 15; general organization, 34-36; Ohio's proposed organization, 92
Cyclopædia of Practical Medicine, introduced by Dunglison, 71; use of bloodletting, 98; recommended physics, 99-100; emetics, 100; tonics, 102; treatment of asthma, 108

Dartmouth Medical School, established, 19
Davidge, John, 58
Davis, N. S., faculty of Rush Medical School, 42; college, 50; educational reform, 78, 93, 94; criticism of strong liquor at American Medical Association meetings, 231; founding of American Medical Association, 237-240, *passim*
Davy, H., 69
Declaration of Independence, Rush signs, 27; signatures and votes of physicians, 171
Degrees (Medical), 13, 15, 17-18 n. 9; number held at outbreak of

the Revolution, 20; term of study, 51-55; ease of attainment, 89-91; attempts to raise requirements, 91-95
Delafield, Edward, Vice-President of the American Medical Association, 240
Delaware (State of), medical regulations, 211 n. 37, 214
Delaware, Medical Society of, 22, 211 n. 37, 214; prizes, 228; history, 228 n. 97
Denman, T., 72
Dental Intelligencer, 185
Dental Register of the West, 185
Dental Surgeons, National Society of, 233
Dentistry, 25; magazines, 185
Devine, Joel, refused admittance to Dutchess County Medical Society, 221
Dewees, W. P., 70, 72; blisters, 101; treatment of croup, 107; treatment of yellow fever, 112; midwifery, 137
Diet, 104, 192
Dissector, asserts its independence, 188
Disinfectants, 102-103
Dissection, requirement of, 49
District of Columbia, see Washington, D. C.
Dix, Dorothea, 117; report to Congress, 126-127, 128-129
Dorsey, J. S., 25, 69
Douglass, Wm., 21
Dover powers, 106
Drake, Daniel, and Medical College of Ohio, 39, 78-81
Drugs, 23; discussion of adulteration of, 192 n. 38; attacks on adulteration of, 229-230
Druitt, R., 69
Dunglison, Robley, 34, 47; author of textbooks, 67-68, 71; criticism of clinical instruction, 89; treatment of constipation, 105
Dutchess County, Medical Society of, refuses admittance to Joel Devine, 221

Earle, Pliny, 122
Eberle, James, 70; treatment of croup, 107; sale of copyright, 179 n. 14

Eclectics, establish college, 41
Eclectic Journal of Medicine, 183
Edinburgh, University of, 13, 19; Rush attends, 26; requirements, 36-37; no American students, 1802, 42; use of Wood's text, 71
Editing, prices, 178-179; methods in magazines, 186-187
Education (Medical), 11; developments, 12, 13-20, 33-95; ethics in, 154; discussions in magazines, 192-193; work of medical societies, 226; summary 243-244; affected by specialization, 246
Ely Resolutions, educational reform movement, 93
Emetics, 23, 26; Sydenham and, 29, 100
Enemas, 105
Ergot, 24, 131-132; discussion in *Medical Repository*, 191
Ether, 141-143
Ethics (Medical), 148-154; enforcement by medical societies, 220-225
Expenses, allowed delegates to meetings of the Medical Society of New York, 219 n. 66
Expulsion, to enforce medical ethics, 221-222
Eye Infirmaries, Cincinnati, 81

Faculties (Medical Schools), powers, 43-44
Febrile diseases, treatment of c. 1770, 26
Fees, medical education, 44, 47-51; reading terms, 51-52; for special medical schools, 53, 151; medical, 154-169
Finley, Reverend Mr., 13, 16, 26
Florida (State of), regulations of medical practice, 213
Fordyce, Wm., 70
Fothergill, John, 16, 64
Fourcroy, A. F., 68
Francis, John W., European study, 43; treatment of Cholera Asiatic, 113, 171
Franklin, Benjamin, 13; loan to Rush, 26, 118
Franklin College, established, 41; fees, 48
Freud, Sigmund, Rush's practices resembles his, 30

INDEX 263

Friends' Retreat (Frankford, Pennsylvania), established, 118; old-fashioned practices, 126
Fyfe, A., 62

Generation, theories of, 130
Geneva Medical College, Elizabeth Blackwell matriculates, 37; established, 40; state appropriation, 45; rowdy spirit, 76-77; hospital attendance of pupils, 89; criticized by Boardman, 90; conditions in study of surgery, 147; seating of representatives at medical society, 236
Georgia (State of), established medical college, 40; regulation of medical practice, 213-214; laws regarding inoculation and free vaccination, 216; revive medical society, 240
Georgia, Medical College of, established, 40; six-month term, 52; proposes national medical society, 237
Georgia, Medical Society of, 1804, 234, 240
Germ theory, 24
Gibson, William, 69
Godman, John D., efforts to publish book, 179
Gonorrhea, 114-115
Gooch, R., 72; case of mother and child, 137
Goforth, William, 78
Good, J. M., 67, 70
Gout, 105-106
Graduation, 74-78
Graham, Sylvester, public diet during Cholera Asiatic epidemic, 113-114
Gram, Johannis B., introduction of homeopathy into the United States, 243
Green, J. C., address on factories, 232
Greene County, Medical Society of, enforcement of medical ethics, 222
Gregory, G., 70; use of bloodletting, 99; treatment of smallpox, 109; treatment of yellow fever, 112; treatment of venereal disease, 115

Gross, Samuel, use of bloodletting, 98; medical charges in Easton, Pennsylvania, 161-162; income, 168, 177 n. 9; remarks on theses, 176; forecast of the medical revolution, 249
Guthrie, Samuel, chloroform, 143

Haggard, H. W., introduction of ergot, 132
Hahnemann, Samuel, homeopathy, 243
Haller, A., 67
Hartford Retreat, 119
Harelip, operation for, 137
Harrison, W. H. (President), 99
Harvard Medical School, 19; attitude of students toward medical co-education, 38; quality of work, 42; relation to University, 43; state appropriation and private endowment, 46; library rules, 73-74; hospital attendance of pupils, 89; rights of graduates to practice, 207
Hayes, Samuel, 165
Hays, Isaac, 148
Health preservation, books on, 179-180
Health regulations, 214-218
Heberden, William, 70
Henry, Patrick, Rush's quarrel with Washington and, 28
Henry, W., 69
Holmes, O. W., 24; contagious nature of puerperal fever, 136; remarks on Bigelow's address, 226
Holten, Samuel, 171
Homeopathy, effect on regular profession, 235; account of, 243
Hope, J., 63
Horner, W. F., 62, 63; advice on dissection, 65-67
Hosack, David, income from private pupils, 34; founds Rutgers Medical College, 83-86; introduction of ergot, 132; reviews of his book, *Febrile Contagion*, 194-195; quarrels in New York City, 236
Hospitals, school hospitals, 89-90; hospitals for the insane, 117-119; ethics in, 149-150; lazarettoes, 214-218

INDEX

Humanitarianism, 127
Hunter, John, 16, 70, 71
Hunter, William, 14, 16; teacher of Rush, 26
Hunter, William (Newport, R. I.), 56
Hydrophobia, 108-109
Hygiene, 145; Percival's advice, 150

Illinois (State of), establishes medical schools, 41; laws permitting dissection, 61; hospital for the insane, 119; regulation of medical practice, 211, 214; revives medical society, 240
Illinois College, established, 41
Illinois, Medical Society of, 211; irregularity of meetings, 235
Illinois Medical and Surgical Journal, 184
Incomes, of physicians, 166-169
Indiana (State of), establishes medical schools, 41; hospital for the insane, 119; medical regulations, 211 n. 37, 214; revives medical society, 240
Indiana, Medical Society of, 211 n. 37; irregularity of meetings, 235; revived, 240
Indiana Medical Convention, censure of clergy, 225
Inoculation, distinguished from vaccination, 109; regulation of, 216
Insanity, Rush's treatment of, 30; 116-129; Percival's advice, 150; progress in treatment, 242
Institutes of medicine (course in), 14
Instruments, in midwifery, 134-135; in surgery, 139-140
Iodine, 24
Iowa (State of), Medical Society, 240
Irregular medicine, 200-203
Ives, A. W., introduction of ergot, 132

Jackson, Charles T., anesthesia, 142
Jackson, Samuel, republication of articles in Europe, 197
Jefferson Medical College, established, 40; quality of work, 42; relation to trustees, 43; state aid to, 46; fees, 48; Drake a professor in, 79; quarrels, 81-82; censured, 86; enrollment, 91
Jefferson, Thomas, remarks on Rush, 171
Jenner, Edward, 24, 109, 110
Journal of Pharmacy, 183
Journal of the Philadelphia College of Pharmacy, 183

Kappa Lambda Society, 233 n. 114; criticism of, 236
Kemper College: see Missouri, Medical Department of the University of
Kentucky, insane asylum, 119
King's College, see Columbia University
Kirkbride, Thomas, 121, 122
Knight, J., President of American Medical Association, 239
Kuhn, Adam, death, 29

Ladies Physiological Institute of Boston and Vicinity, 233 n. 114
Laennec, R. T. H., auscultation, 241
Lavoisier, R. L., 68-69
Laws (Medical), 22; attitude of public, 42; Virginia, law of 1736, 155, 204-218
Laxatives, 99-100
Lee, Arthur, 171
Lee, R., 72, 130; use of forceps, 134; cæsarian section, and abortion, 135
Leeches, 197
Lewis, Winslow, 71
Lewis, Winslow, Jr., advice on dissection, 65-67
Libraries, of medical colleges, 73-74; medical societies, 226-227
Liquor, anesthetic use of, 141
Liston, R., 69
Literature (Medical), 11; early publication, 20-21, 174-200; reviews, 193-195; summary, 244-245
Lobelia leaves, 201-202
Lockrow, V. B., barred by Albany Medical Society, 222
Long, Crawford, anesthesia, 142
Lottery, to raise funds for the Medical Department of the University of Maryland, 45; use in Kentucky, 46
Louisiana (State of), appropriation for medical education, 46; hospi-

INDEX 265

tal for the insane, 119; medical charges, 163-164; medical regulations, 212; free vaccination, 216

Louisiana, Medical Department of University of, faculty, 39; established, 40; state appropriation, 46

Louisiana Medical and Surgical Journal, 185

Louisville Journal of Medicine and Surgery, 183

Louisville, Medical Institute, established, 40; quality of its work, 42; relation to trustees, 43-44; city endowment, 45; boarding house rates, 50; Drake a professor in, 79; quarrel with Transylvania, 86; enrollment, 91

Manley, Beck and McCall, proposals for educational reform, 93

Macquer, P. J., 68

Magazines (Medical), 11, 12, 21; educational news, 47-48, 181-199; summary, 245; specialization in, 247; effect of cheap publication, 248

Magendie, F., 67

Maine (State of), laws permitting dissection, 61; hospital for the insane, 119; regulation of medical practice, 208, 214; free vaccination, 216

Maine Medical College, see Bowdoin College

Maine, Medical Society of, 208; irregularity of meetings, 235

Manning, Thomas, introduction of vaccine into America, 110

Maryland (State of), post-mortem, 57; insane asylum, 119; medical regulations, 211 n. 37, 214

Maryland Hospital for the Insane, use of restraining apparatus, 124, 125

Maryland, Medical Department of the University of, established, 38-39; trustees and regents, 44; state appropriations, 45-46; fees, 48; requires dissection, 49; term of study, 51

Maryland, Medical and Chirurgical Faculty of 211 n. 37; rules for library, 227

Massachusetts (State of), laws permitting dissection, 59, 60-61;

Worcester Hospital, 119; regulation of medical practice, 204-208, *passim*

Massachusetts General Hospital, insane department, 117, 118-119; use of patent medicine, 224

Massachusetts Medical College, see Harvard Medical School

Massachusetts Medical Society, 22; rates for apprenticeship in Essex South District, 33; required readings, 62, 63; pharmacopœia, 71; publication, 175-176, 206-208, 218-240, *passim*

Materica medica, 14; Rush's attitude, 30; study of, 71-72; changes, 104

McClellan, George, founds Jefferson Medical College, 40, 54

McDowell, Ephraim, ovariotomy, 138

McLean Hospital (Department for the Insane of the Massachusetts General Hospital), 118-119

M'Naughton, James, 171; founding of American Medical Association, 238

Medical jurisprudence, study of, 72

Medical Repository, 21, 181-182; objects of the magazine, 190-191

Meigs, C. D., 72; attitude towards puerperal fever, 136

Memphis Medical Institute, established, 41

Menstruation, 101

Mercury, use of, 102

Mesmerism, anesthetic use, 141

Michigan (State of), insane asylum, 119; medical regulation, 214

Michigan, Medical Department of the University of, established, 41; reform of curriculum, 88

Midwifery, 16; Shippen's work, 16-17; professorship, 56; textbooks, 72, 96, 129-137

Mifflin, Thomas, 111

Mississippi (State of), hospital for the insane, 119; medical charges, 163-164; medical regulations, 211 n. 37

Mississippi, Medical Society of, 211 n. 37

Missouri (State of), establishes medical schools, 41; laws per-

mitting dissection, 62; medical society, 240
Missouri, Medical Department of the University of, fees, 48; established, 41
Mitchill, John, influence on Rush's treatment of yellow fever, 31
Mitchill, S. L., 21; *United States Pharmacopœia*, 72, 171, 181
Monro, Alexander, 62
Moral treatment (of the insane), 117-118, 124-125
Morgan, John, plan for education, 13; sketch, 13-15, 22, 27, 28
Morphia, 24
Morton, C. T. G., anesthesia, 142
Mott, Valentine, European study, 45; translation of Velpeau, 70, 138-139, 139-147, *passim*
Murray, J., 71; physics, 99; emetics, 100; tonics, 102; lithontriptics, 103

Narcotics, 105
Nationalism, in medical journals, 196-197
Negroes, use in dissection, 62
Newell, Mark, restored to Connecticut Medical Society, 223
New England Journal of Medicine and Surgery, 182
New Hampshire (State of), laws permitting dissection, 61; hospital for the insane, 119; medical regulations, 211 n. 37; requires vaccination, 216
New Hampshire, Medical College of: see Dartmouth Medical School
New Hampshire Medical School, established, 22; control of education, 44; educational reform movement, 92; *Police*, 149, 211 n. 37
New Haven County, Medical Society of, first publication, 175
New Jersey (State of), law permitting dissection, 60; medical charges, 162; medical regulations, 206, 211 n, 37, 214; free vaccination, 216-217
New Jersey Asylum for the Insane, model construction, 120-121; rules for attendants, 124; host to Dorothea Dix, 129

New Jersey, Medical Society of, established, 22; first fee table, 156, 211 n. 37; organization, 218
New Orleans, Medical Society of, 233 n. 114
New Orleans Medical and Surgical Journal, 184-185
New Orleans, Physico-Medical Society of, 233 n. 114
New York (State of), appropriations for medical education, 45; laws permitting dissection, 60, 61-62; post-mortem, 57; Utica Asylum for the Insane, 119; number of physicians, 1831, 166; medical legislation, 205-206, 209-211; free vaccination, 216-217; laws during cholera epidemic, 217; quarrels within the profession, 236
New York Academy of Medicine, 232-233
New York City, difficulties of profession, 18; quarrels, 119; British occupation of, 18 n. 10; anatomical riot, 57-58; hospital for the insane, 119; medical fees, 156; 1816, 158-159 ff.; Vaccine Institute, 216-217; advertising for patent medicines, 203; regulation of medical practice, 205-206; medical quarrels, 236
New York County, Medical Society of, 22; relation to the College of Physicians and Surgeons, 44, 82; investigation of patent medicines, 203; libraries, 227; social activities, 231-232
New York Dispensary, Medical Association of, 233 n. 114
New York City, Physico-Medical Society of, 233 n. 114
New York Hospital, insane department, 117, 119
New York, Medical Department of the University of the City of, established, 19, 41; quality of work, 42; state appropriations, 45; boarding house rates, 47, 50; aid to impoverished students, 48; short-courses, 52, 85; enrollment, 91
New York, Medical Society of, report on terms of study, 51-52; educational reform movement, 92,

93; ethics, 152-153; family contracts, 165, 209-211; 218-240 *passim*
New York Medical and Philosophical Journal and Review, 182
New York Society for the Relief of Widows and Orphans of Medical Men, 233 n. 114
North American Archives of Medical and Surgical Sciences, 183
North Carolina (State of), hospital for the insane, 119; medical society, 240
North Carolina, Medical Society of, 234
Northwestern Medical and Surgical Journal, 184

Ohio (State of), act to protect graves, 59; hospital for the insane, 119; medical regulations, 211-212
Ohio Asylum for the Insane, use of restraining apparatus, 124-125
Ohio, Medical College of, established, 39; relation to trustees, 43-44; state grant, 46; professors, 56; salary of Samuel Gross, 168
Ohio Medical Convention, 75; educational reform movement, 92, 212; organization, 218
Ohio Medical Repository of Original and Selected Essays and Intelligence, 185
Oliver, D., 68
Oneida County, Medical Society of, expulsion of member for performing abortion, 222
Onondaga County Medical Society, 93
Opium, anesthetic use of, 141

Paine, Martyn, attack on proposed Medical Convention, 238
Paresis, first described, 122
Parrish, Joseph, 166
Patent medicines, 203; expulsion from medical societies for their manufacture, 222-223; use in Massachusetts General Hospital, 224; endorsed by clergy, 225; proposals by Alabama Medical Convention, 229
Patterson (N. J.), Vaccine Institute, 216-217

Paxton, J., 63
Pennsylvania (State of), constitution, 27; aid to Jefferson Medical College, 46; medical society, 240
Pennsylvania College for Homeopathy, established, 41
Pennsylvania Hospital, 16, 64; library, 73; insane department, 117, 119
Pennsylvania Hospital for the Insane, moral treatment, 125
Pennsylvania Medical College, established, 41
Pennsylvania, Medical Department of the University of, history, 13-17, 18; requirements, 35; students in attendance c. 1800, 38; quality of work, 42; fees, 48; graduation fee, 49; cost of education, 50-51; six-month term, 51; enrollment, 91
Percival, Thomas, 148-152
Pereira, J., 72
Perkins, Elisha, Patent Metallic Tractors, 200-201, 222
Philadelphia (City of), medical fees, 159-160; residence of medical authors, 178
Philadelphia, College of, history of, 13-17; merged with University of Pennsylvania, 28
Philadelphia College of Pharmacy, Code of Ethics, 152
Philadelphia College of Physicians, 23; Rush's resignation from, 31; library, 73; proposals to Governor of Pennsylvania for prevention of yellow fever, 111-112; medical charges, 160; dues, 219, 232
Philadelphia Journal of Medical and Physical Sciences, 182
Philadelphia Medical College, established, 41
Philadelphia Medical Museum, 182
Philadelphia Medical Society, 153
Philadelphia Monthly Journal of Medicine and Surgery, 182-183
Phlogiston theory, 68; discussion in *Medical Repository*, 191
Physical education, 192
Physicians and Surgeons of the City of New York, College of, history of, 17-18; requirements, 35; established, 38-39; trustees,

44; state appropriations, 45; fees, 48; dissection room, 49; six-months term, 51; library, 73; graduate course, 77; reaction to salaried professors, 87; quarrel, 82-85
Physicians and Surgeons of the Upper Mississippi, College of, established, 41
Physicians and Surgeons of Western New York, College of, established, 39; ceases operation, 41; boarding-house rates, 50, 54; attitude towards "body-snatching," 58; cadavers, 60; division of fees among professors, 86-87
Physick, P. S., 53; treatment of cuts incurred during dissection, 65; bandaging in surgery, 146-147
Physics, 99-100
Physiology, Rush teacher of, 29; study of, 67-68
Pierce, Daniel, 165
Pinel, Philip, Rush's importance, 30-31, 116, 127, 128
Pleurisy, treatment c. 1770, 26
Post, Wright, European study, 43
Post-graduate School, surgery and midwifery, 77
Post-mortem, 57
Potter, N., bloodletting, 99
Practice of Physick, 96-147; few changes, 242; specialization, 246-247
Preceptor, 33, 54
Prescriptions, character, 103
Prizes, awarded by medical societies, 227-228
Professorships, 55-56; specialization in, 246
Puerperal fever, 11, 24, 136
Pure Foods and Drugs Act, 230
Purges, 23, 26; Sydenham's use of, 29, 99-100

Quacks, treatment of tuberculosis, 106; Percival on, 151; attitude of the public, 154; books by, 202-203; medical societies attempt to control, 224; effects on regular physicians, 242-243
Quain, J., 64
Quarrels (Professional), in medical schools, 78-79, 81-86; Percival's advice on, 151

Ramsey, David, 21, 22; author, 172
Ramsbotham, F. H., 72
Ray, Isaac, 129
Reading term, use in New England, 52-53
Redman, John, 14, 26
Reform, educational, 91-94
Regents of the University of the State of New York, 18; relation to education, 44; quarrel in College of Physicians and Surgeons in New York City, 82-86
Revolutionary War, Rush's part, 27-28
Rheumatism, treatment of, c. 1770, 26, 106
Rhode Island (State of), free vaccination, 216; law during the cholera epidemic, 217
Richerand, A., 67
Rigby, E., 72; midwifery, 134; cæsarian section, 135
Riots, anatomical riots, 57-58, 59
Roget, P. M., 68
Romayne, Nicholas, 18
Rush, Benjamin, 20, 21, 25-32, 70; advice to graduates, 76; use of bloodletting, 97; treatment of tuberculosis, 106-107; treatment of hydrophobia, 109; yellow fever, 112; cholera infantum, 114; insane, 117-118; importance in history of psychiatry, 128; ethics, 148, 149; advice on charges, 155-156; Jefferson's letter to Adams, 171
Rush Medical College, established, 41; quality of its work, 42
Rutgers Medical College, 19, 82-86, 210

St. Louis Medical Institute, established, 41; professors, 56
Salaries, of professors, 42; at College of Physicians and Surgeons of Western New York, 86-87; proposals for reform, 86-87; of staffs of insane asylums, 121; physicians to penitentiaries and jails, 168; of health officers, 215
Sarbin, L. B., expelled from Massachusetts Medical Society, 222
Scarifying, 97-98
Seaman, Valentine, course for midwives, 130; preceptor of Valentine Mott, 138

INDEX

Sedatives, 105
Select Medical Library, 183
Semmelweiss, 24; contagious nature of puerperal fever, 136
Shattuck, George, income, 169
Shaw, J., 63, 65
Shippen, William, Jr., 13, 16-17, 26; quarrel with Rush, 27-28; riots of 1765, 57, 64
Silliman, Benjamin, Jr., 69
Simms, Marion, operation for vesico-vaginal fistula, 138
Simpson, J. Y., chloroform, 143
Sloughter, Governor, post-mortem on, 57
Smallpox, 109-111; health regulations regarding, 216-217
Smellie, W., 72
Smith, E. H., 111
Smith, N. W., expelled from Medical Society of Oneida County, 222
Societies (Medical), 12, 21-23; control of medical colleges, 44; educational reform, 78; aid in establishing insane asylum, 129; publications, 175-176, 204-240; summary, 245
Society of Medical Superintendents and Physicians of Hospitals and Asylums for the Insane, 129, 233
South Carolina (State of), insane asylum, 119; medical charges, 162-163; medical regulations, 211 n. 37, 214; revives medical society, 240
South Carolina, Medical College of, established, 40; ceases operation, 41; term, 51; quarrel, 85
South Carolina, Medical College of the State of, takes over Medical College of South Carolina, 40; quarrel, 85
South Carolina Medical Association, see South Carolina Medical Society
South Carolina, Medical Society of, 211 n. 37; censure of clergy, 225; library, 226; removal of unsatisfactory drug inspector, 230; revived, 240
Southern Journal of Medicine and Pharmacy, 185
Southern Medical and Surgical Journal, 183-184; attempt to found national medical association, 237
Spalding, Lyman, *United States Pharmacopœia*, 71-72; introduction of ergot, 132
Specialization, in surgery, 147; in magazines, 198, 246-247
Stahl, G. E., p. 25
Starling Medical College, established, 44; endowment, 46
Stearns, John, treatment of croup, 107; introduction of ergot, 132
Sterility, cause and treatment, 131
Stevens, A. H., introduction of ergot, 132; ligating, 145-146
Stewart, F. C., number of practitioners, 91
Stillé, Alfred, Vice-President of the American Medical Association, 240
Stimulants, 102
Stokes, William, 71
Strychnine, 24
Subscription, rates of magazines, 188-189
Summer lectures, 50
Sumner, George, 96-97
Supreme Court, invalidates regulatory law of Washington, D. C., 211
Surgeon-General, Library of, 73
Surgery, 24-25; fees for course, 48; textbooks, 69-70, 138-147; summary, 241-243
Sweating, 23, 26, 101
Sweat, William, 165; income, 169
Sydenham, Thomas, effect upon Rush, 29, 70; prescription by, 103; treatment of: gout, 105-106; tuberculosis, 106; hydrophobia, 108; smallpox, 109; confusion of gonorrhea and syphilis, 114
Symes, James, 69
Syphilis, 114-115; as a cause of insanity, 122

Temperance, Percivals' advice on, 151; movement, 228, 230-231
Tennessee, laws permitting dissection, 61; hospital for the insane, 119; revives medicial society, 240
Tennessee, Medical Society of, irregularity of meetings, 235; revived, 240

Texas (State of), medical regulations, 213
Textbooks, 62-64, 65, 67-72
Thatcher, Thomas, 20
Theory and Practice of Medicine (course in), 14; Rush professor of, 29; study of, 70-71
Theses, 75; Gross's remarks on, 176
Theory (Medical), 11-12, 24; "system," 25; Rush, 26-31, 96-97; general, 131
Thomas, R., 100; confusion of gonorrhea with syphilis, 114
Thomsonians, Society, 202; right to practice in Alabama, 212; status in Georgia, 213; affect upon reguprofession, 235
Thomson, Samuel, satire on allopathic treatment of insanity, 122-123, 201-202
Ticknor, Luther, 167
Tonics, 23, 102
Transylvania University, Medical Department of, established, 39; quality of its work, 42; relation to trustees, 43-44; lottery for, 46; publishes magazine, 41-48; fees, 48; library, 73; length of thesis, 75; Drake, 78; quarrel with Louisville, 86
Treasurer of the United States Mint, Rush's appointment, 31-32
Tremont Street School (Boston), 53
Tuberculosis, 106
Tuson, E. W., 65
Tweedie, William, 70-71

United States Pharmacopœia, 71-72, 176
Utica, Hospital for Insane, 119; practices, 125-126; publication of journal, 185

Vaccination, 24, 78, 109-111; of babies, 137; encouraged by states, 216-217
Vaccine Inquirer, 183
Vaccine Institutes, New York City and Patterson, N. J., 216-217
Van Buren, Martin, 171
Vegetable diet, Rush's use in yellow fever, 31; interest in, 242
Velpeau, A. A. L. M., 69-70; relations with V. Mott, 139

Venereal disease, 114-115; Percival's advice on cases of women, 150; soliciting business in, 224
Venesection, 97
Vermont (State of), laws to protect graves, 59; hospital for the insane, 119; medical regulations, 211 n. 37
Vermont Academy of Medicine, see Castleton Medical School
Vermont, Medical College of the University of, established, 39-40; control of education, 44; attitude towards "body-snatching," 58; cost of cadavers, 65, 85-86
Vermont Medical Society, attempt at educational reform, 92, 211 n. 32
Virginia (State of), insane asylum at Staunton, 119; regulation of medical fees, 155; regulation of medical practice, 204, 213; free vaccination, 216
Virginia, Eastern Asylum of, 118
Virginia, Medical Department of the University of, established, 40; Richmond branch, 40-41; state appropriations, 46; term, 51-52; professors, 56

Warren, John, 26; Boston fee table, 156
Warren, John Collins, anesthesia, 141-142; average day of, 172-173; on physical education, 179-180; support of Graham's dietary reforms, 224
Warren, Joseph, 26
Washington College of Baltimore, established, 40
Washington, D. C., Medical Association of, fees, 160-161
Washington, D. C., Medical Society of, 211, 214; library, 227
Washington, George, Rush's quarrel with, 27-28
Waterhouse, Benjamin, vaccination, 110; endorses Thomson's system, 201; position in Massachusetts Medical Society, 223
Watson, John, 94-95
Watson, R., 68
Watson, Thomas, 71
Webster, J. W., 69
Wells, Horace, anesthesia, 141

INDEX

Western Journal of Medical and Physical Sciences, 183
Western Journal of Medicine and Surgery, 183-184
Western Medical and Physical Journal, 183
Whooping cough, 108
Willard, Elias, expelled from Albany Medical Society, 222-223
Willoughby University, Medical Department of, established, 40
Winer, Andrew, expelled from Greene County Medical Society, 222
Winslow, J. B., 62
Wistar, Caspar, 62, 63
Wisconsin (State of), establishes medical school, 41
Wisconsin State Medical Society, 234
Women in medicine, 37-38; colleges for, 41
Wood, G. B., 71; and Franklin Bache, 72; treatment of croup, 107; treatment of Cholera Asiatic, 114

Woods' Quarterly Retrospect of American and Foreign Practical Medicine and Surgery, 185
Woodstock Medical College, established, 40; fees, 48; examination fee, 49; boarding-house rates, 50; beginning of the term, 54
Woodward, Samuel, 122
Worcester Asylum, 119
Worcester District Medical Society, library, 226
Worthington, Robert, account of Berkshire Medical Association, 234-235
Wyman, Rufus, 129

Yale College, Medical Department of, established, 39; relation with medical society, 44; fees, 48; aid to poor students, 49; relation to Medical Society, 208; negotiations with Connecticut Medical Society, 225-226
Yellow fever, Philadelphia epidemic 1793 and Rush, 31-32; treatment of, 111-112; interest in, 191

Bei Fragen zur Produktsicherheit wenden Sie sich bitte an:
If you have any questions regarding product safety,
please contact:

Walter de Gruyter GmbH
Genthiner Straße 13
10785 Berlin
productsafety@degruyterbrill.com